WEEK L

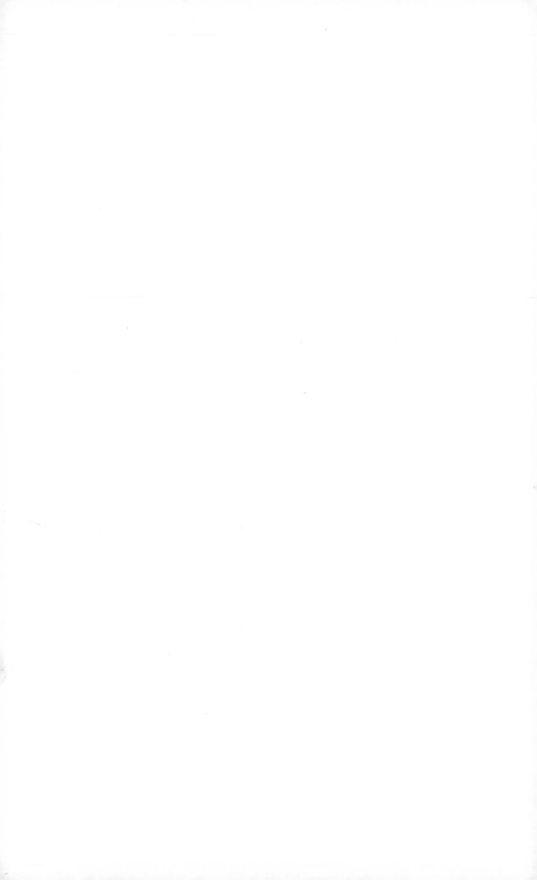

Mild Head Injury

Mild Head Injury
a guide to management

PHILIP WRIGHTSON

lately Neurosurgeon

and

DOROTHY GRONWALL

lately Neuropsychologist

Concussion Clinic, Department of Neurosurgery,
Auckland Hospital, Auckland, New Zealand

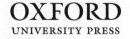

OXFORD
UNIVERSITY PRESS

OXFORD

UNIVERSITY PRESS

Great Clarendon Street, Oxford OX2 6DP

Oxford New York

Athens Auckland Bangkok Bogotá Buenos Aires Calcutta
Cape Town Chennai Dar es Salaam Delhi Florence Hong Kong Istanbul
Karachi Kuala Lumpur Madrid Melbourne Mexico City Mumbai
Nairobi Paris São Paulo Singapore Taipei Tokyo Toronto Warsaw

and associated companies in
Berlin Ibadan

Oxford is a trade mark of Oxford University Press

Published in the United States
by Oxford University Press, Inc., New York

© P. Wrightson and D. Gronwall, 1999

The moral rights of the authors have been asserted

A catalogue record for this title is available from the British Library

Library of Congress Cataloging in Publication Data
Wrightson, Philip.
Mild head injury / Philip Wrightson and Dorothy Gronwall.
Includes bibliographical references and index.
1. Concussion.   2. Brain damage.   I. Gronwall. D. M. A.
II. Title
[DNLM: 1. Brain Injuries–diagnosis.   2. Brain Injuries–therapy.
WL 354 W9545m 1999]
RC394.C7W75 1999   617.4'81044–dc21   99-19511
ISBN 0 19 262939 5

Typeset by Downdell, Oxford
Printed in Great Britain
on acid-free paper by
Biddles Ltd,
Guildford and King's Lynn

Preface

For some 25 years we have been concerned with the investigation and management of the problems which can follow mild head injury, and for the past 15 years have run a clinic for people affected by them. Over this time we have seen a remarkable change in attitudes. When we started, many of our colleagues thought that most if not all of the complaints of the 'post-concussion syndrome' were neurotic or even dishonest. We believe that there is now a fairly wide acceptance of an organic basis for them. There is more understanding that any process such as this which affects our thinking, emotions, and judgement, the most intimate part of our existence, must generate secondary emotional changes. It is becoming recognized that these are usually a result and not a cause of the syndrome, and that their management is an important part of treatment. It has become appreciated too that the family, friends, workmates, and employers are also involved and are often ignorant and judgemental, as once many of us were, and need to be informed and persuaded to help.

Management therefore needs a variety of skills. Neurology and neuropsychology provide the first assessment and follow-up, followed by clinical psychology, social work, and counselling. Later the apparatus of vocational assessment and job finding may be necessary. Questions of compensation are important and there must be effective cooperation with lawyers and administrators. Separate referral to each discipline is tiring for the patient and time consuming and wasteful in other ways. We think it is important therefore not only to bring all these disciplines together in the same place, but to try to unite them into an interdisciplinary team. Everyone then understands the other member's job, does a little of it themselves, but knows their limitations and when to call in expert help.

We have tried to write this book as a guide to people who want to take part in running such a service for those with head injuries. We have taken them to be expert in their own field, though not necessarily in its application to mild head injury. We hope that the book will provide a special point of view and help practitioners to deal with the neurological, cognitive, and behavioural problems that so often follow mild head injuries. It may also help in dealing with the similar problems met with in the more severely injured.

Written by a neuropsychologist and a neurosurgeon, the book may be lacking in other areas of expertise and we hope that practitioners in these areas will be generous and forgive our simplicity. We have tried to remedy some of the deficiencies by consulting colleagues, and we are very grateful indeed to Dr Jonathan Simcock, Dr Greg Finucane, and Dr Ian Civil for their help; Mr Charles N. Simkins has generously helped us with comments on litigation in the United States.

We would like to thank all the others who have helped us over the years to make this concept work. In particular, those who have worked in the clinic as part of their training and as research assistants, particularly from the Department of Psychology of the University of Auckland, and from the Department of Psychiatry at Auckland Hospital. We are much indebted to the Medical Research Council of New Zealand and to the New Zealand Neurological Foundation for financial support, and to Auckland Hospital for acceptance of our clinic.

Not least we would like to say how grateful we are to the hundreds of people who have attended our clinic over the years and have taught us about the many facets of mild head injury, and who have given us so much feedback about what does and what does not help them to deal with their problems.

Note on 'Further reading'

At the end of each section we have suggested some further reading. These mostly refer either to the original observations, particularly when these are of interest in the development of thinking on the subject, or to papers which supply further technical details. As far as possible these have been chosen from publications likely to be available in most medical libraries.

As well as this there are several books dealing with more general aspects of the recovery from head injury which can be recommended to readers, listed below.

1. Ponsford, J., Sloan, S., and Snow, P. (1995). *Traumatic brain injury: rehabilitation for everyday adaptive living.* Lawrence Erlbaum Associates, Hove.
   A 'hands-on' but scholarly book, written by clinicians with an extensive experience of head injury rehabilitation. Though not specifically concerned with the mildly injured population, it has many sections that are relevant to their problems.
2. Richardson, J. T. E. (1990). *Clinical and neuropsychological aspects of closed head injury.* Taylor & Francis, London. (2nd edn. in press 1999.)
   An excellent review and analysis of the literature up to the time of publication, for those who wish to research the field in detail. It covers head injury of all degrees of severity, not just mild injury.
3. Gronwall, D., Wrightson, P., and Waddell, P. (1998). *Head injury – the facts: a guide for families and care-givers*, (2nd edn). Oxford University Press, Oxford.

This was written primarily for patients and their families and, though it is concerned with head injuries of all severities, it has sections addressed specifically to patients with mild injuries.

4. King, N. (1997). Mild head injury: neuropathology, sequelae, measurement and recovery. *British Journal of Clinical Psychology,* **36**, 161–84.
   An excellent review of recent literature covering many aspects of mild head injury assessment and rehabilitation.

Contents

List of abbreviations

ASD   acute stress disorder
CI   confidence interval
CNP   canalith repositioning manoeuvres
CNS   central nervous system
CSF   cerebrospinal fluid
CT   computed tomography
DSM-IIIR   *Diagnostic and Statistical Manual of Mental Disorders –*
   Version IIIR
DSM-IV   *Diagnostic and Statistical Manual of Mental Disorders –*
   Version IV
ED   emergency department
EEG   electroencephalogram
GCS   Glasgow Coma Scale
ICD   International Classification of Diseases
MHI   mild head injury
MR   nuclear magnetic resonance (scan)
fMR   functional MR
NSAID   non-steroidal anti-inflammatory drug
PASAT   Paced Auditory Serial Addition Test
PCS   post-concussion syndrome, symptoms
PET   positron emission tomography
PTA   post-traumatic amnesia
PTSD   post-traumatic stress disorder
RA   retrograde amnesia
RTA   road traffic accident
SPECT   single photon emission computed tomography
TBI   traumatic brain injury
TENS   transcutaneous electrical nerve stimulation

1

Introduction

This chapter describes the development of the present concepts of the mechanisms and results of mild head injury. The sequence of organic changes, cognitive impairment, and the reaction to disability is outlined. Early management is important and there is a need for a service that can deal with problems before they become entrenched.

Mild head injury can be defined in a number of ways. Lay people see it as a minor event followed by rapid and complete recovery. In fact in the acute stage there is the possibility of life-threatening complications, and later disabling somatic and cognitive problems may persist and behavioural problems develop. In both cases there is the paradox of an apparently trivial event resulting in an illness with major consequences. The acute complications result from physical processes and are easy to understand. The later problems depend on the relation of brain structure to thinking and behaviour, and are still a matter of some controversy.

The writings of the ancient Egyptians and Greeks show that they were used to treating wounds of the head, and knew of the risk of acute complications from apparently trivial injuries. Medical writing since then has continued to describe this immediate risk. Only in the last 200 years has much been said about symptoms which may occur later. Hilton, writing in the mid 1800s (Hilton 1877), in his *Lectures on Rest and Pain*, describes changes in the personality and the ability to concentrate on business in a man of substance who was concussed after a fall from his horse. He recommended that he should rest as much as possible and work strictly within the limits of fatigue. Texts in the early 1900s describe late symptoms following concussion and suggest that they could be treated by rest and general health measures; when these were ineffective it was likely that the patient was 'neurasthenic' – weak in character and with little will to get better. Later the experience of mental breakdown in two wars and the awareness of stress reactions to trauma made it easier to ascribe persisting symptoms of mild head injury to neurosis rather than to physical damage.

As physiological psychology developed it was used to examine cognitive function after head injury. Ruesch in 1944 (Ruesch 1944) devised tests of speed and thought and fatiguability, and suggested that there were abnormalities after head injury. In 1958 Dencker and Lofving reported a study of identical twins, where one of each pair had had a head injury three years or more earlier. They found that though there were no differences between the pairs on standard intelligence tests, the twins that had had a head injury performed less well in tests of attention and reaction time.

At the time, however, the tests remained research procedures and did not lead to studies of patients in the clinical situation, looking at their progress over time and seeing how tests related to the other symptoms that they reported.

There were also differences in opinion on what was meant by a 'mild' head injury. Traditionally the occurrence of coma and its duration had been used, together with the duration of amnesia, both retrograde, covering the events before the injury (RA), and post-traumatic amnesia (PTA) covering those afterwards. There was disagreement whether it was necessary for there to have been a definite loss of consciousness or whether a period of confusion or amnesia would be sufficient. There were those who would define mild head injury in terms of a post-traumatic amnesia of less than an hour, and others who would accept a period of up to 24 hours. Possible resolutions are discussed in Chapter 2.

Amongst clinicians views on the nature of these symptoms differed widely. In 1962 Sir Charles Symonds, in a classical paper, pointed out that since the 1940s there had been good pathological evidence of neuronal damage after concussion, and suggested how retrograde and post-traumatic amnesia could be explained, and how some cognitive processes might remain impaired. Repeated minor injury could be expected to cause progressive loss. Symptoms which persisted were due in part directly to this structural damage and in part to the patient's reaction to the impairment it caused.

Writing in the same period a sharply contrary view was expressed by Henry Miller (1966). He maintained that symptoms were rare when there was no claim for compensation, as in sports injuries, and that their apparent severity was inversely proportional to the duration of unconsciousness and amnesia that was claimed. There were no signs of an organic basis. Persisting symptoms were due to 'accident neurosis' or frank malingering and disappeared when claims were settled. It is fair to say that his views depended largely on assessments of claims for compensation after industrial accidents, not sports or other injuries, and that physicians with a similar practice today have some sympathy with them.

By 1970 clinicians caring for patients who had problems after a mild head injury had to take their stance somewhere between that of Symonds or Miller, with no physical signs to go by and no reliable test procedures to guide them. Many patients certainly were anxious and depressed, and perhaps most clinicians felt that these were the important features and treated the patient with counselling and antidepressants.

Those who did not respond again tended to be labelled as neurotic or malingerers.

The first major prospective clinical and psychological study was published in 1974 by Lidvall, Linderoth, and Norlin. A group of patients were followed for 3 months after a mild head injury, using a battery of cognitive and behavioural tests and studying electroencephalograms (EEGs) and vestibular function. Three months after injury a quarter were still complaining of significant symptoms. However, the authors could find no consistent relation between the results of their tests of cognitive function and their measure of the severity of the injury and concluded that the symptoms were related to depression, anxiety, and poor motivation, without an organic basis. Unfortunately their measures of severity, their 'organic basis', was their estimate of the duration of PTA. The way they determined this would not now be accepted as reliable, and their use of three grades out of four within a PTA duration of less than an hour, on which their comparison depended, is unrealistic. Further, as will be seen in Chapter 3, PTA is only one of the possible indices of organic damage.

The situation changed when it was established that the psychometry which had been used up to that time was not necessarily sensitive to the effects of minor head injury. In 1974 the use of the first practical test of the impairment of cognitive function was described, the Paced Auditory Serial Addition Test (PASAT) (Gronwall and Wrightson 1974). It was shown to give a measure of the ability to concentrate and attend, and to process information. In fit young men who had been concussed the PASAT score was significantly lower than normal in the first fortnight or so but had returned to the expected level by 35 days after the accident. Later studies showed that in an unselected group of patients admitted to hospital a similar temporary reduction was found, but that test scores remained low beyond this time in the small proportion in which clinical symptoms persisted. Since this time PASAT has come to be widely used as a basic measure of information processing capacity after head injury, as a serial measurement to chart recovery and as a practical index of readiness for normal work.

The relation of the clinical symptoms to the cognitive defects that had been demonstrated by these and other tests became plainer over the next few years. Studies of an unselected population with mild head injury by Rimel et al. (1981) and of a sub-section of young physically fit men by the authors (Wrightson and Gronwall 1981) showed that there was a group of symptoms which was common to the great majority of people in the early days after mild head injury. They were present at all ages, whether there were claims for compensation or not and people injured at sport were not exempt, as Miller and others had claimed. In some cases these early symptoms continued, with the reaction to them varying according to their severity and to the personality and circumstances of the victim, as would the response to any threat. The patient's state then depended on the sum of the direct effect of injury and the reaction to it, and their recovery on the separate resolution of each of these two factors. Sometimes the reaction might continue when the direct effect had recovered, resulting in a chronic disability.

Since these early clinical studies the basic neuropsychology of mild head injury has been investigated extensively and the effects on memory, perception, and organization and their interrelation described. New imaging techniques have allowed these changes to be related to structural damage, particularly in the temporal and frontal lobes. It has become possible to distinguish and understand a variety of different clinical pictures associated with the neuropsychological changes and to adjust management to suit them.

Several important issues have emerged. It has been shown that even when there has been apparently complete recovery mild head injury can result in a lasting impairment (Gronwall and Wrightson 1975). It may not be detectable under ordinary circumstances, but becomes apparent under conditions of stress such as hypoxia. This is illustrated by a study of two groups of university students, the members of one of them having made a full functional recovery from a mild head injury occurring more than two years earlier. They were tested both at normal atmospheric pressure and at a simulated altitude of 12 500 feet in a hypobaric chamber. There was no difference between the groups at ground level, but the students of the head injury group performed at a significantly worse level when they were mildly hypoxic (Ewing *et al.* 1980). Slight impairment of capacity of this sort may become significant in people with highly demanding jobs. Like the students they do well on standard tests, and it may be difficult to explain why their performance at work has lost its edge.

Though there may seem to be complete recovery from one injury, further concussions can increase the impairment to the point that it becomes clinically significant. This is a major issue in sports injuries and it has been important to convince the management of sporting bodies that there is a need to make rules to protect players from long term damage.

Mild head injuries are common in young children. It has been thought that late effects were rare, but now it seems possible that there may be slight and perhaps significant impairment of development of reading and other skills. One study followed two groups of pre-school children who had had accidents and been taken to hospital emergency departments (EDs) but had not needed admission. Members of one group had had a mild head injury, the other a laceration or minor orthopaedic condition. There was no difference between the groups in the scores of neuropsychological tests in the first few weeks after the accident, but by 12 months children of the head injury group scored significantly below the others on some visual tasks, and when they were seen at the age of $6\frac{1}{2}$ years, more of the head injured group had needed help in learning to read (Wrightson *et al.* 1995).

In many emergency departments mild head injury is now managed efficiently and safely, using formal protocols for procedures and relying on CT scans when complications are suspected. In many places patients discharged from hospital wards and emergency departments are told about the symptoms they may encounter during recovery and how to get advice if they persist. Often, however, this system fails, as patients are pushed through the system as fast as possible. Most emergency departments are not geared to long term follow-up, neurological and neurosurgical services have more acute and demanding cases to attend to, and psychiatric services may not be appropriate in the earlier stages and later referral to them may not be acceptable to the patient. As a result some patients with problems receive little effective management until their condition is chronic and established and treatment has become more difficult. In some centres, however, the need has been recognized, and special clinics have been set up in which patients can be seen soon after the injury, a diagnosis and assessment made, and rehabilitation and support arranged. The organization and work of clinics of this sort is one of the major concerns of this book.

References

Dencker, S. J. and Lofving, B. (1958). A psychometric study of identical twins discordant for closed head injury. *Acta Psychiatrica Neurological Scandinavica*, **33** (Suppl.), 122.

Ewing, R., McCarthy, D., Gronwall, D., and Wrightson, P. (1980). Persisting effects of minor head injury observable during hypoxic stress. *Journal of Clinical Neuropsychology*, **2**, 147–55.

Gronwall, D. and Wrightson, P. (1974). Delayed recovery of intellectual function after minor head injury. Lancet, **ii**, 605–9.

Gronwall, D. and Wrightson, P. (1975). Cumulative effects of concussion. *Lancet*, **ii**, 995–7.

Hilton, J. (1877). *Lectures on rest and pain*. (2nd Edition) George Bell & Sons, London.

Lidvall, F., Linderoth, B., and Norlin, B. (1974). The causes of the post-concussional syndrome. *Acta Neurologica Scandinavica*, **20** (Suppl.), 56.

Miller, H. (1966). Mental effects of head injury. *Proceedings of the Royal Society of Medicine*, **59**, 257–66.

Rimel, R. W., Giordani, B., Barth, J. T., Boll, T. J., and Jane, D. A. (1981). Disability caused by minor head injury. *Neurosurgery*, **9**, 221–5.

Ruesch, J. (1994). Intellectual impairment in head injuries. *American Journal of Psychiatry*, **100**, 480–96.

Symonds, C. P. (1962). Concussion and its sequelae. *Lancet*, **i**, 1–5.

Wrightson, P. and Gronwall, D. (1981). Time off work and symptoms after minor head injury. *Injury*, **12**, 445–54.

Wrightson, P., McGinn, V., and Gronwall, D. (1995). Mild head injury in preschool children: evidence that it can be associated with a persisting cognitive defect. *Journal of Neurology, Neurosurgery and Psychiatry*, **59**, 375–80.

2
Definitions and epidemiology

Introduction

Mild head injuries make substantial demands on health services. They take up a good deal of time in EDs, and they may need expensive imaging and sometimes short term use of hospital beds. Later a small proportion of patients have persisting symptoms which keep them off work for long periods and require costly rehabilitation and disability pay. For both economic and clinical audits it is important to know how many injuries there are, how they are managed and why, and for how long patients are disabled.

However, there are problems in defining what is meant by mild head injury. Plainly it is part of a continuum extending from injuries that are trivial to those which threaten life. Where we place the marker which separates the 'mild' injury from a severe one will depend on our needs and interests. Those responsible for the organization of accident services and EDs will see a mild head injury as one in which the patient loses consciousness, recovers rapidly with only supportive treatment, and needs minimal hospital care; later events will not be taken into account. Other clinicians may be concerned with patients who originally met these criteria but now complain of disabling symptoms. Again, some patients exhibit these same symptoms after an injury which was obviously more severe. Plainly there cannot be a single definition which covers all these situations. One has to be used which meets the needs of the moment, and it must be kept in mind what its limitations are.

Most epidemiological studies have been concerned with the factors important in providing for the early management of milder injuries. For this purpose the distinction between these injuries and those that are more severe has been made in several ways. It is most satisfactory to employ clinical criteria, and those most often used have been the level of consciousness when first seen, and the duration of PTA. In a large scale audit there are, however, practical problems if definitions of this sort are used, as they require the analysis of individual case notes. A simpler approach may be sufficient, using hospital statistics and International Classification of Diseases (ICD) codes, identifying a diagnosis of simple head injury and, if possible, confirming it by either discharge home from the ED or a short admission to hospital.

Most studies have depended on hospital contacts. Many mild injuries, however, are treated outside hospitals by private emergency clinics or general practitioners. In some communities the number of such patients is considerable, and of the same order as the number of patients seen at hospitals.

It is also important to include the substantial number of patients who have been admitted to hospital primarily for other injuries but who also have had a head injury. These can be identified in a formal audit of case notes and classified by the duration of unconsciousness and the length of PTA. As before, it may be more practical to identify them in hospital discharge statistics, provided the coding for secondary injuries can be relied upon.

Determining the incidence of later problems is difficult. Many people have unpleasant symptoms for several weeks or months after mild injuries. These symptoms may not be sufficiently severe or disabling for patients to seek medical advice but if they do they may consult one of a variety of doctors, general practitioners, neurologists, or others. Tracing them, making sure that their problems are indeed due to head injury and recording data for a retrospective study, is rarely practical. If there is a clinic with a special interest in head injury, data from a sufficient number of these patients may be collected and it may be possible to extrapolate and to get some idea of the incidence.

Prospective studies have been done on groups of patients, identifying them in EDs and following them for several months or a year. Patients have usually reported a high incidence of symptoms, but often it has been uncertain whether the subjects would have complained if they had not been asked, how disabled they were, and what was the contribution of litigation. A major difficulty is that in such prospective studies it has been practical only to include a limited number of subjects. If the incidence of cases with persisting problems is of the order of 5 per cent, as it appears to be, the size of the sample needs to be very large in order to detect any significant differences in incidence even when they are present.

In this chapter we will suggest practical definitions of mild head injury and its complications, and present data on its epidemiology from the literature and our own experience.

Definition of mild injury

A practical definition of mild head injury is needed which serves two purposes. Emergency departments need to define, classify and count the patients they treat. Later, in the assessment of persisting problems it is useful to know how severe the original injury was.

The definition needs to be in two parts. The first is a minimal standard, specifying that there has been a disturbance of neurological function. This is necessary because about half the people coming to EDs with an injury to the head show no sign of this. The second part describes an upper limit of severity, separating cases in which there are focal neurological abnormalities, significant brain damage seen on imaging, or slow recovery from the acute symptoms.

Definition of minimal severity

(1) The history from the patient or an observer indicates that there has been an injury to the head resulting from physical force.

(2) The injury disturbed neurological function, with one or more of the symptoms of confusion, amnesia, or alteration of consciousness, either immediate or delayed; or there may have been other events of neurological significance such as severe and persistent headache or vomiting without other explanation.

This definition is made when the patient is first seen. It does not depend on reports of duration or depth of unconsciousness and it accepts that other symptoms of neurological impairment may be present when there has been no loss of consciousness. It covers the delayed onset of symptoms seen in children, and the delayed development of amnesia after minor injury (see Chapters 3 and 4).

Definition of an upper limit of severity

The second part defines an upper limit of severity, separating mild injuries from those that are 'moderate' or 'severe'. This assessment may be made when the patient is first assessed, on their state after an initial period of observation, or on discharge if they have been admitted to hospital.

Grading of severity at first assessment

When first seen patients with a mild injury should have a Glasgow Coma Scale (GCS) score of no less than 13. There should be no major focal neurological abnormalities such as hemiparesis or cranial nerve damage.

This definition has the advantage of using a familiar and well authenticated scale, but the rating will depend on the interval between the injury and assessment. In general a score of 15 is a reliable indication of a mild injury, though an occasional patient will deteriorate later. Those with a score of 13–14 are likely to improve, but some will remain at this level and be classed as having a more severe injury or will deteriorate because of complicating pathology.

An example of data gathered on arrival is an epidemiological study by Kraus and Nourjah (1989), which selected patients with a GCS score of 13–15 at or shortly after arrival in the ED, and who were admitted to hospital. Looking at the outcome, this population included 5.4 per cent of subjects with gross brain lesions (ICD 851–853) and 14.4 per cent with 'other intracranial conditions', (ICD 854), some of which would also have been serious. Again, 36 per cent needed to stay in hospital for more than three days. Plainly, though many of these subjects had suffered an injury which, on the single criterion of the GCS score, was labelled as mild, their progress in the next few days placed them in a different category.

A second study of those with a GCS score of 13–15 is that of Dunham *et al.* (1996) in which routine CT scans showed that there was a significant incidence of intracranial haemorrhage, mostly when there were soft tissue injuries of the upper face and scalp. (See Chapter 4.)

Grading after initial observation

Common practice in EDs is to observe patients for a period, usually around 4 h, before deciding on further care. Patients with a GCS score of 15 and no complicating factors may be suitable for home management. Though the guidelines for admitting patients to hospital vary from place to place and with time, these can be graded as mild head injuries. Studies of this large group have been made in Scottish EDs (Strang *et al.* 1978) and by the authors (Wrightson and Gronwall 1998).

If the CGS score does not improve to 15, or if there are other risk factors, observation in hospital is usual, with grading deferred until this period of observation is completed.

Grading on discharge from hospital

Most patients who have been admitted to hospital for observation will improve over the next 24–48 h. Those that are discharged within this period will be graded as having mild head injuries. The remainder will be excluded. Grading becomes difficult if there is a need to include those whose discharge is delayed because of other injuries. They may be identified from the clinical record of GCS scores and neurological state, or by the duration of PTA; this may not be practical in an ordinary epidemiological study.

An example using these criteria was the study by Rimel *et al.* (1981). This specified a history of unconsciousness of 20 minutes or less, a GCS score of 13–15 on arrival at the ED, and less than 48 h hospital admission. None of the patients deteriorated after discharge.

From the evidence of the first two of these reports, it is plain that selection by the level of consciousness alone includes conditions too severe to be classed as mild head injury. The added criterion of no more than two days in hospital is clinically simple and easy to use in a survey.

Later assessment of the initial severity of head injury

When a patient is seen weeks or months later their account of the symptoms that they had and how they were treated will usually be enough to
determine whether their condition in the first 48 h or so corresponds
with the definition of mild head injury we have given above. The duration
of PTA is important in confirming this. If it is not evident from the history it can be estimated by asking the patient for an account of the events
before and after the injury, and defining the end of PTA by the time when
his memory of events became continuous, being careful to distinguish
'islands' of recall. It must be cautioned, however, that later estimates
made in this way do not always correspond well with those made in the
ED and during admission to hospital (Gronwall and Wrightson 1980).

Some have made PTA the principle criterion of the severity of the
injury, proposing that mild head injury should be defined by an upper
limit of 24 h. As an example, Alexander (1995) proposes that in mild
head injury 'confusion with amnesia ... is present by definition for less
than 24 hours, but usually for minutes to a few hours'. In Table 1 we give
the PTAs of a group of patients with mild head injury who had been sent
home from the ED or who had been admitted to hospital for less than
48 h. Plainly the definitions by management and by PTA correspond
well.

For the clinician the definition by PTA is attractive, as it reflects the
patient's condition. However, it requires the examination of case notes
and becomes impractical when many cases are being surveyed.

Patients with head injuries admitted for management of other injuries

Many patients who are admitted to hospital with an orthopaedic or trunk
injury have also had a head injury. This may be severe and a major factor

Table 1 Post-traumatic amnesia in patients either
admitted for two days or less or treated at home

PTA	Number	Percentage
0–5 min	90	50
6–60 min	37	20
1–6 h	33	18
7–24 h	15	8.5
1–7 days	6	3.5

Source: authors' data.

in the outcome, but is often mild. These patients are not included in most accounts of mild head injury, but they provide a significant number of referrals for long term effects. The clinical findings at the time of admission may be clear enough to classify the injury as mild, and the PTA determined retrospectively will be important. However, both estimates may be invalidated in more severe injuries by analgesia or anaesthesia.

Patients managed entirely outside hospital

We will see later that a considerable number of head injuries are treated by private clinics or general practitioners. In all classifications these patients would be regarded as having had mild injuries.

The incidence of mild head injury and of late complications

Sources of information

Plainly the most reliable method is a prospective study in which the investigators examine ED and hospital inpatient data as each patient presents, make sure that they fit the criteria, and then follow the patient to recovery. There will be the usual epidemiological difficulties: a single ED may give a biased sample, the community from which they are drawn may not be representative, there may be significant seasonal variations, and several departments may need to be surveyed. When the incidence of late effects is to be studied substantial numbers, of the order of several thousands, will be needed.

A less costly method is to search the hospital data published by health administrations. Admissions with the ICD rubrics of 850 and 854 are reasonably likely to be of patients with mild head injuries; if the definition used allows a skull fracture, some of ICD 801 may be acceptable. The results will, however, depend on the accuracy of the coding. If the data available include duration of hospital stay, the selection of cases admitted for two days or less will make the results more certain.

In some places coded data are available on patients seen in ED and sent home. However, if the individual notes are not examined it may be uncertain whether the minimal criteria for a mild head injury were present. A further group which may be overlooked in ED data are those in which other injuries were more important and the head injury was incidental.

Some people with mild head injuries are not seen in hospital but are treated by general practitioners or private emergency clinics. There is no practical way of making a direct count of these, though it may be possible to estimate them from the number of patients who present later with persisting symptoms.

Lastly, population surveys such as the United States National Health Interview Survey can give an estimate of the number of people who report that they have had a head injury, whether it was treated medically or not (Sosin *et al.* 1996).

Statistical methods

The incidence of head injury will usually be given as cases per hundred thousand of the whole population per year. There is a difference in incidence between males and females and between those in the 15 to 35 age group and those at the young and old extremes of life. When these differences could be important it is better to give incidences in 100 000 of the target group, rather than to the total population. Again, comparisons between incidences in other places should be made with caution, as there may be significant differences in population distributions.

Source of statistics and methods

The statistics that follow are from two studies by the authors (Wrightson and Gronwall 1998). They were collected with the problems of managing mild head injury in mind, particularly those of the later effects. We have compared them with data from other sources when this has been possible.

The first study is of some 2500 hospital contacts occurring over an eight week period in 1986. They occurred in Auckland, New Zealand, a seaport and manufacturing city with a well defined population at the time of 850 000. The patients were seen first at the EDs of the four general hospitals serving the city. At the time of the study the great majority of medical consultations for acute head injury took place at the EDs of these hospitals, so that the statistics are likely to give an accurate picture of head injury in the area. Whether the conclusions are applicable to other cities on the basis of size, location, ethnic composition, and sports participation needs to be considered, but the figures do compare reasonably well with those in studies made elsewhere.

The second study is a survey of patients seen in the five years 1990 to 1994 in a clinic run by the authors for people with cognitive and behavioural problems following head injury. The area from which patients came was the same as that covered by the first survey, and though there is an interval between the two studies, it is thought reasonable to relate them to each other.

Incidence and policies of management

Table 2 gives the incidence of mild and more severe head injuries with neurological symptoms seen in the four EDs, classified by their management. Those in hospital for up to two days and those not admitted have

Table 2   Cases seen in emergency department with definite neurological symptoms: cases per 100 000 of whole population per year

Disposal	Age 0–14		Ages 15+		All ages	
Not admitted	229		425		654	
Admitted as primary head injury						
Days in hospital						
0–2	23		11.5		34.5	
3–7	5.4		9.2		14.6	
8+	4.6		11.5		16.1	
Total		33		32.2		65.2
Total with mild injury	252		437		689	
Admitted for treatment of other injuries	14		43.6		57.6	
Total[†]	276		501		777	

* Disposal: admitted, not admitted, and primary treatment.
† Based on a total of 1015 cases of head injury with neurological symptoms.
Source: authors' data.

been counted as mild injuries. How many of those with other injuries were in this class is not known, but data from the second study suggest that it is likely to have been two out of three.

Only a small proportion of the patients with mild injuries were admitted to hospital – 9 per cent in the under 15s and 2.6 per cent in the older group. It is important to be aware that this proportion varies from place to place, so that figures for admission alone do not give a true incidence. Table 3 illustrates this, comparing data from Auckland and San Diego, a seaport and city of similar size. The incidence of major injuries was almost identical, but four times as many patients with mild injuries were admitted.

Policies on admission for mild injuries depend on the confidence that ED staff have in their diagnosis, the availability of inpatient beds for observation of doubtful cases, and on the local medicolegal requirements. They may change with time. In New Zealand the annual admissions for milder head injuries with ICD codes 850 and 854 over ten years fell from 8517 to 4985, whilst those for more severe injuries with codes 851–853 rose from 204 to 315. The factors in this change were the availability of

Table 3 Incidence of admissions to hospital for head injury in Auckland and San Diego, expressed as admissions per 100 000 total population for three durations of hospital stay

Hospital stay (days)	Auckland, 1986	San Diego, 1981
0–2	34.5	131
3–7	14.6	15
8	16.1	14
All stays	65.2	160

Source: Authors' data and Kraus and Nourjah 1989.

CT scans, which were able to rule out major pathology, and increased pressure on inpatient beds.

Not all mild head injuries are seen at hospital EDs. Cases treated by private emergency services and general practitioners are likely to be less severe, but they do result in temporary disability and time off work, and some have persisting problems. In the authors' clinic 40 per cent of the patients referred because of persisting symptoms after mild injuries had been treated by general practitioners only. This proportion is comparable with the findings of the National Health Interview Survey in the USA for 1991 which found that 40 cases of head injury had been medically treated outside hospital for every 100 seen in EDs and discharged home (Sosin *et al.* 1996). The incidence of cases of all ages not admitted to hospital, $618/10^5$/year, is close to that in New Zealand, $654/10^5$.

Age and causes of mild head injury

Figure 1 shows the variation of the incidence of mild head injury with age. In the first five years the numbers are high, due to falls occurring in young children. It rises again at 15 and reaches a peak in the early 20s with road traffic accidents, and then declines in the 30s and remains low.

Further information on the causes at various ages is given in Table 4, which gives the incidence related to the numbers in each age group in the population. Notable features are again the number of falls in the 0–4 age group, with a high proportion of admissions, and the large number of cases in the 15–34 year age group, dominated by minor road accidents.

Incidence of persisting symptoms after mild injuries

In the first of the authors' two studies, 566 patients aged 15 and over who had neurological symptoms were not admitted to hospital, and of these

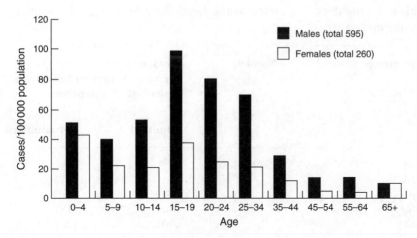

Fig. 1. Patients seen in emergency departments with mild head injury and discharged for management at home, expressed as cases per 100 000 whole population per year. Source: authors' data.

27 were referred to their clinic because of persisting symptoms, an incidence of 4.9 per cent (95 per cent CI 3–7). Of the 72 cases of mild injury which were admitted to hospital, seven were referred (9.7 per cent, 95 per cent CI 4–19). In 60 per cent of the patients the referrals were made more than 28 days after the injury, indicating that the complaint was more than trivial. In the second study there were 242 referrals of patients aged over 14 who had had mild injuries, out of an estimated 18 000 cases over five years, an incidence of 1.3 per cent (95 per cent CI 1–2).

These figures illustrate the problems of obtaining an accurate count of the incidence. The first study was prospective, made under well controlled conditions, and included at total of 2500 cases, but the number with persisting symptoms after mild injury was small and the confidence intervals wide. In the second study the authors' clinic was only one of a number of agencies to which patients could be referred, and the incidence appeared to be substantially less than that in the first study.

Considering the data available, 1.3 per cent would be likely to be a significant underestimation, and an incidence of the order of 3 per cent for referrals after 28 days would appear to be reasonable.

Factors in referrals for persisting symptoms

It is of interest to know whether persisting symptoms are commoner in men or women or as a result of particular injuries. As an estimate the numbers involved in various categories of accidents in the first study were compared with the referrals in the second.

Table 4 Incidence of injury to the head with neurological symptoms, by age and cause

Age group (years)	Number	Incidence/100 in age group per year: injury to head with neurological symptoms	
		Admitted	Not admitted
0–4	319		
RTA		50	111
Falls		140	909
Others		100	187
Total		290	1207
5–9	211		
RTA		50	248
Falls		90	317
Others		9	237
Total		149	802
10–14	212		
RTA		104	268
Falls		10	236
Sport		8	364
Others		17	43
Total		139	911
15–34	1038		
RTA		88	978
Falls		16	88
Sport		14	200
Assault		25	195
Others		9	84
Total		152	1545
35+	328		
RTA		36	82
Falls		13	64
Sport		2	11
Assault		5	40
Others		9	27
Total		65	224

Cases from eight weeks' survey of four EDs.
Source: authors' data.

In accidents where there had been falls, objects striking the head accidentally, and assaults there was no difference in the male/female proportion. In sporting injuries, however, females were referred more often than men, as was the case with minor traffic accidents.

Similar comparisons were made with age groups. There was a tendency for the 15–24 age group to be less likely to complain of symptoms, only significant in the case of assaults and sports.

There was no difference in the proportion of cases referred after road traffic accidents, assaults, or sports injuries, and people injured in falls were significantly less likely to complain. People injured by accidental blows were, however, more likely to complain, perhaps because these injuries tend to be sustained at work and the elements of fault or compensation are often involved.

The interval between accident and referral with persisting symptoms

The interval between accident and referral is of interest in giving some idea of the period of disability and of the state of service for patients. Data from the authors' clinic are given in Table 5. In most cases the referral was the first to a specialist facility. The greatest number was first seen between four and 16 weeks after the injury, but a significant number had not obtained specialist help a year or more later. These data of course reflect a local situation, and in other places referral may be swifter and more effective. They do, however, suggest that doctor education ranks with provision of facilities as an important factor in the management of these people.

Table 5 Interval between accident and specialist referral: cases treated initially by GP, by hospital ED, and not hospitalized, and by ED and admitted to hospital for two days or less

	Interval (days)				
Treated by	**0–28**	**29–112**	**113–365**	**365+**	**Median**
GP	17	34	16	9	53*
ED	35	51	22	16	57*
ED and admitted	5	11	8	5	100
Total	57	96	46	30	
% of Total	25	42	20	13	

* Difference in medians not significant.
Source: authors' data.

Summary

Mild head injury is part of a continuum ranging from the trivial to the mortal injury. There is no natural division of the upper limit of its severity and this may be chosen to suit the use that is to be made of it.

For the purposes of epidemiology a practical way of defining mild head injury is in terms of management. Patients should have shown a definite disturbance of neurological function due to mechanical injury and they should have been managed at home or admitted to hospital for not more than two days. This definition includes the significant group treated only by general practitioners.

Further clinical criteria may be added. A GCS score of 13–15 when first seen may be required, though this depends on the time of examination. There should be no major focal neurological signs. The duration of PTA, determined in the acute stage or later, is the most important addition; when this is defined as being up to 24 h it corresponds well with the definition by management.

It is important not to rely on hospital statistics only. The proportion of people with mild injuries admitted to hospital has fallen steadily over the past ten years, with the availability of CT scanning and the pressure to keep patients out of hospital beds. A significant number of injuries are treated by general practitioners outside hospital.

The incidence of mild head injury in the population aged 15 or over is around $500/10^5$ of whole population/year, and of those under 15 around $275/10^5$/year, but the age-specific incidences show a higher figure for the younger group of $2900/10^5$/year compared with $1770/10^5$ for the older.

The major causes of injury in the under 15s are falls, with road traffic accidents and sports following. In the 15 to 34 group road accidents are by far the commonest cause, with sport and assaults some way behind. Road accidents and falls are the causes in the 35 and upward patients.

There is a higher incidence of all injuries in the 15 to 34 age group, peaking in the 20–24 interval. Females are less often involved than males.

The incidence of persisting symptoms needing specialist consultation is around 3–5 per cent. Women are a little more likely to be referred after traffic accidents and sports injuries, but the rates are otherwise equal. People injured by accidental blows to the head are more often affected, but the rates for other injuries do not differ. In particular, men injured in sport are not less liable to persisting symptoms than others.

By the time patients are referred for specialist advice they have often been restricted by symptoms for many months; the economic cost is therefore considerable, and it is important that there should be effective identification and management of these people.

References

Alexander, M. P. (1995). Mild traumatic brain injury; pathophysiology, natural history and clinical management. *Neurology,* **45**, 1253–60.

Dunham, C. M., Coates, S., and Cooper, C. (1996). Compelling evidence for discretionary brain computed tomographic imaging in those patients with mild cognitive impairment after blunt trauma. *Journal of Trauma, Infection and Critical Care,* **41**, 679–86.

Gronwall, D. and Wrightson, P. (1980). Duration of post-traumatic amnesia after mild head injury. *Journal of Clinical Neurophysiology,* **2**, 51–60.

Kraus, J. F. and Nourjah, P. (1989). The epidemiology of mild head injury. In *Mild head injury,* (ed. H. S. Levin, H. M., Eisenberg, and L. M. Benton). Oxford University Press, New York.

Rimel, R. W., Giordani, B., Barth, J. T., Boll, T. J., and Jane, J. A. (1981). Disability caused by minor head injury. *Neurosurgery,* **3**, 221–8.

Sosin, D. M., Sniezek, J. E., and Thurman, D. J. (1996). Incidence of mild and moderate brain injury in the United States, 1991. *Brain Injury,* **10**, 47–54.

Strang, I., MacMillan, R., and Jennett, B. (1978). Head injuries in accident and emergency departments in Scottish hospitals. *Injury,* **10**, 154–9.

Wrightson, P. and Gronwall, D. (1998). Mild head injury in New Zealand: incidence of injury and persisting symptoms. *New Zealand Medical Journal,* **111**, 99–101.

3
Mechanisms and pathology

Introduction

The mechanical factors in mild head injury and the cellular pathology that follows have been difficult to unravel. Human studies, of necessity, have been limited to clinical observation and to the imaging and neurophysiological studies that have been ethically justifiable, with occasional autopsy material available from people who have had a mild head injury and have died from other causes. Experimental injury in subhuman primates has worked out the important mechanical factors and some of the pathology, but the model is an expensive one and there have been ethical difficulties, so that its usefulness is probably over. More recent experimental work has used small animals such as rats, with injury by fluid percussion or similar methods rather than gross mechanical forces, and with this model it has been possible to gain considerable insight into the cellular and chemical processes.

In many areas detailed explanations are yet to come, but there is often enough to throw at least some light on the events which matter to the clinician. Those to bear in mind in the account which follows are

(1) the immediate loss of consciousness with injury;
(2) delayed effects – the later drowsiness of small children and the delay in onset of retrograde and post-traumatic amnesia;
(3) the lack of uniformity in the clinical picture, particularly of the relations between the occurrence and duration of coma and cognitive loss;
(4) the sensitivity to further injury;
(5) the cumulation of loss with repeated injury; and
(6) abnormalities in imaging, particularly those of perfusion.

Experimental models

In the early years of the century investigators tried to reproduce the features of human head injury by subjecting a variety of animals to a direct impact on their head, usually with the head not free to move. A blow of sufficient force to produce coma usually resulted in gross brain damage, and recovery from this was unusual. In 1941 Denny-Brown and Russell established that temporary coma and recovery could be produced by accelerating a freely mobile head. In the next 30 years there were many similar experimental studies, especially in monkeys, as animals with a brain anatomy similar to that of humans. It proved difficult, however, to imitate human concussion, with its temporary loss of consciousness, full recovery, and absence of obvious lesions in the brain. Eventually with refinement of the mechanical systems it was possible to show that in primates, controlled acceleration in the sagittal plane could imitate human concussion, with microscopic damage only. A similar acceleration in oblique and coronal planes produced a longer period of coma, but there tended to be macroscopic lesions, especially in the corpus callosum and superior cerebellar peduncles (Gennarelli *et al.* 1982).

In the 1980s the technique of fluid percussions was developed for investigating both severe and mild injury. A small area of dura is exposed and a watertight connection made to a column of fluid. A pulse of pressure in the fluid is transmitted through the dura to the brain. Others have produced a similar pulse by a transient mechanical impact such as a falling weight. The damage to brain tissue caused by these pulses closely resembles that produced by head acceleration in primates. With its use of small animals and simple apparatus this has become the preferred method for investigating fine structural and chemical changes (Foda and Marmarou 1994). These are probably very similar to those occurring in humans, but differences in gross anatomy and neural circuitry make the method less relevant to human problems such as the impairment of consciousness, vascular reactions, and late effects.

Pathological anatomy in mild head injury

In 1959 Strich described damage to axons after severe head injury, and in 1968 Oppenheimer showed that this could be seen at autopsy of people who had suffered only a mild head injury and died from other causes. Since then more powerful staining methods have made this easier to demonstrate. It had originally been thought that the axonal sheath was torn across at the time of the injury, usually where it changed direction or hooked round a vessel, and that axoplasm flowed out to form the 'retraction balls' that are typical of the histological picture. Recent work has shown that the first event after injury is an infolding of the axolemma and alteration of neurofibrils, with an accumulation of organelles proximal to this. Only after an interval of hours or even days does the axonal sheath rupture and release the disorganized contents to form the typical ball (Povlishock and Christman 1995). The extent to which this change has progressed can give an estimate of the length of survival after the injury.

Damage to cell bodies as well as to axons can be seen in experimental mild injury. This may result in cell necrosis with inflammatory changes, or in apoptosis, where the cell disappears without this reaction. With newer staining techniques dendrites can be seen to be affected. Petechial haemorrhages also occur in mild injury, though they are not a prominent feature. Changes in small vessels may be more important. In severe injuries these changes are well documented, and they are likely to occur to a lesser extent in mild injury. There is swelling of the astrocytic foot processes, changes in the endothelium over some distance, and disruption of the blood–brain barrier.

Chemical changes in mild head injury

It has long been known that neuronal injury leads to the release of a variety of neurotransmitters such as glutamate which result in a cascade of further toxic cell damage. This can occur as a result of mechanical stress without gross deformation, such as occurs in the fluid percussion model of MHI. After injury there is an immediate depolarization, with an influx of sodium and calcium ions and a large increase in extracellular potassium ions and then of various neurotransmitters. Especially in sensitive areas such as the hippocampi, cell death occurs, with either necrosis or apoptosis as mentioned above (Hayes and Dixon 1994). Where the blood–brain barrier is affected, circulating excitotoxins may gain access to neurons and increase the damage.

Changes responsible for coma

Because of the concept that consciousness depends on the reticular activating system, it was at first taken that damage to this system was the cause of the immediate loss of consciousness after head injury. In the 1980s evidence began to accumulate that this was not the case, and that it was probable that a brainstem inhibitory system depending on muscarinic cholinergic transmission was responsible (Hayes and Dixon 1994); at a second stage other excitatory amino acids would accumulate, prolonging the effect and possibly leading to long term damage.

The evidence for this concept, derived from animal studies but still without confirmation in the human case, is as follows.

(1) The EEG changes. In lesions of the reticular activating system there are generalized slow waves, whereas after concussion there is fast activity (11–23 Hz).

(2) Stimulation of the dorsal brainstem between the collicular and mid-pontine levels produces an acute suppression of EEG activity similar to that seen when consciousness is lost in concussion. The stimulus may be electrical or produced by the injection of cholinergic compounds such as carbachol.

(3) There is evidence of immediate depolarization in this (and other) areas, with large increases of the concentration of potassium ions in the earliest stages and of neurotransmitters slightly later.

(4) Acetylcholine antagonists such as scopolamine reduce the duration of coma.

Delayed and transient effects

Clinical studies of amnesia in the period immediately after injury have shown that it takes some minutes for both pre- and post-traumatic amnesia to be established. In a study in which footballers were tested immediately after a mild head injury there was at first good recall of what had happened before the accident; retrograde amnesia then developed after a few minutes (Yarnell and Lynch 1970). Another study examined the occurrence of 'islands' of recollection during a period of post-traumatic amnesia. These were almost all in the first quarter of the period, suggesting that it took some time for recall to be blocked (Gronwall and Wrightson 1980). In Chapters 4 and 11 we describe the delay which occurs in the onset of symptoms in children who have been concussed. Plainly the injury has set in motion processes which are much slower than the one responsible for the initial loss of consciousness. Several explanations have been offered. It may be that a chain of chemical changes has been initiated that needs time for development before it can inhibit neuronal function. The anatomical basis of the amnesia is presumably the hippocampal cells of the temporal lobes, which are specially sensitive to trauma and hypoxia.

In the case of the delayed onset of symptoms in children a part may be played by a disturbance of perfusion; this may be mediated by a trigeminovascular reflex, for sensory stimulation in the trigeminal area can be shown to produce cerebral hyperaemia with the release of vasodilatory peptides (Sakas and Whitwell 1997). A similar reflex may be responsible for the acute attack of migraine which may occur after a blow to the head, typically in football or boxing. When the attack is severe, consciousness may be lost and the condition can then be confused with concussion (see Chapter 6, footballer's headache, and Chapter 12). However, unlike concussion, there is complete resolution of symptoms within 24 h and no persisting cognitive defect. The way in which consciousness is impaired in these two syndromes is uncertain, but it would appear to be different from the usual mechanism of concussion.

The lack of uniformity in the clinical picture

Definitions of what constitutes a mild head injury commonly use the length of coma and the conscious level when first seen, together with the duration of post-traumatic amnesia, implying that these three quantities march together. This is certainly the case with duration of coma and the GCS score when first seen, as they are plainly aspects of the same state. Although the duration of PTA shows a general relation to these measures there are frequent discrepancies, most often with the duration of PTA being longer than would be predicted from a short period of coma. Indeed, there may be a period of PTA when there has been no loss of consciousness. A further disparity exists in the relation between PTA and the clinical state of confusion. In the recovery stage after concussion it is common for the patient to be lucid but still in PTA.

MR studies examining the location of lesions and relating them to the duration of coma and PTA have shown that the number of lesions in central brain structures correlates with both the duration of coma and PTA, but that the hemispheric damage, in particular to temporal lobe structures, correlates with PTA only (Wilson *et al.* 1994).

In a similar way the variations in the pattern of neuropsychological impairment in MHI indicate that different areas of brain have been affected; with the wide variation in the force and direction of impact this would be expected. As the severity of the injury increases more of the possible sites of injury are taken up, and the pattern then becomes more uniform from case to case.

Sensitivity to repeated injury

The clinical features of the major and minor syndromes of second injury are described in Chapter 12. In the rare major syndrome the second mild injury occurs within a fortnight of the first and is followed in less than an hour by deep coma, usually with death within 24 h. Imaging shows gross brain swelling; at autopsy this is confirmed and usually there is some cerebral contusion or subdural bleeding, but less than would be expected. In some cases there has been evidence of mild inflammation with perivascular cuffing, and a recent history suggesting a viral illness. The most likely explanation is that the swelling is due to a rapid and uncontrollable generalized cerebral hyperaemia, perhaps mediated through the trigeminovascular system. Localized areas of hyperaemia can certainly be demonstrated by single photon emission CT (SPECT) imaging in the first ten days or so after a mild injury, and perhaps these predispose to the catastrophic onset of generalized hyperaemia.

The minor syndrome is often seen when a patient who is showing persistent symptoms after a mild injury suffers a further quite trivial injury, and at once their condition reverts and sets their recovery back by several weeks; a similar setback may occur after a general anaesthetic. It is possible that in areas where there has been excitotoxic damage the process can easily be reactivated, or that areas of hypoperfusion may be sensitive to further mild injury. There is no definite evidence for either explanation.

The cumulation of loss with repeated injury

It is well known that people who have been concussed a number of times – rugby footballers and boxers in particular – change in character and lose some of their abilities. There is also good evidence that lasting but subtle changes can persist even after single minor injuries. In Chapter 1 we referred to the deterioration in some aspects of cognitive performance which was produced by mild hypoxia in a group of university students who had been concussed a year or more previously. Again, we showed that recovery from a second concussion is slower than that after the first. There is therefore good clinical evidence of cumulation.

Cognitive changes can also occur when there has been no actual loss of consciousness, as in whiplash injuries. The deterioration seen in professional boxers is another example, where the cause appears to be the number of bouts fought rather than the number of knockouts (see Chapter 12).

The pathological evidence for cumulation is necessarily indirect. There is no doubt, however, that in single mild injuries there is damage to axons, and probably to cell bodies with necrosis or apoptosis and to microvasculature; further injuries must compound this loss.

Changes seen in clinical imaging

Structural changes – CT and MR scans

Major changes such as substantial cerebral contusions or intracranial haemorrhage would not be consonant with MHI. Other MR abnormalities are, however, commonly seen. They are present mostly in the grey matter, particularly in the frontotemporal areas, with smaller lesions in the major tracts such as the corpus callosum and internal capsule (Levin *et al.* 1992). The correspondence between these areas and histological changes has not been adequately described in humans. Presumably there are the various degrees of cell necrosis and apoptosis seen in experimental animals, together with changes in the neurons whose axons have been severed.

Changes in perfusion

After MHI, SPECT scans often show localized abnormalities in perfusion (see Chapter 7). There are areas of underperfusion which are substantially more frequent than the MR abnormalities, and when both techniques have been used in the same patient there is little correspondence between the location of the abnormalities in MR and in SPECT. The underperfusion may indicate areas where neuronal function is depressed and metabolism reduced, but where the structural changes are not sufficiently great for them to be shown on MR. It is also possible that the perfusion may be reduced by damage to the vascular endothelium. The abnormalities tend to disappear over a matter of months, but in one study 10 per cent were still present after a year, with some correlation with the persistence of symptoms (Jacobs *et al.* 1996). Areas of hyperperfusion are sometimes found, usually close to but not congruous with MR abnormalities; usually they disappear after ten days or so. They may be related to susceptibility to the major second injury syndrome.

Impairment of autoregulation is an important factor in major head injury; it has been described in mild injury but does not appear likely to be significant (Jünger *et al.* 1997).

Correlation of pathology with clinical features

Returning to the features listed in the introduction:

1. The immediate loss of consciousness in MHI is probably best explained by the cholinergic brainstem inhibitory mechanism. It is probably not the cause of continued coma, which may be due to other structural damage, probably to the reticular activating system.

2. In adults the interval which occurs before the onset of retrograde and post-traumatic amnesia is likely to be due to the time taken for chemical changes to occur in the hippocampal areas. The delay on onset of drowsiness in children may be due to a reflex hyperaemia, though the direct evidence for this is slight. Alternatively, as in adults, it may represent the time taken for a cascade of chemical changes to develop, presumably in the brainstem. It is not evident why the process should be different from that in adults.

3. The lack of uniformity in the effects of mild head injury in humans reflects the variability of the lesions in primate experiments, where the location of damage depended on the direction and magnitude of the acceleration. Lesions in the brainstem affecting consciousness and in the cerebrum with cognitive effects occur independently. Only when the injury is severe and most of the possible sites of damage have been affected does the picture become uniform.

4. The sensitivity to a further injury in the major syndrome seems likely to be due to a vascular reaction; this may be mediated through the trigeminovascular system. In the minor syndrome it is probable that abnormal areas, either those shown by MR or by hypoperfusion in SPECT, are sensitive to further trauma or chemical disturbance so that lesions which are healing are reactivated.

5. The cumulation of loss seems to be well explained by damage to axons and by the areas of neuronal necrosis or apoptosis that have been demonstrated in mild injury.

6. MR shows changes mostly in the cortex which could represent areas of cell damage. There are persistent areas of hypoperfusion which correlate with symptoms, though not with MR changes. Other vascular changes – impaired autoregulation and the trigeminovascular reflex – may be responsible for delayed coma in children and migraine-like phenomena.

References

Denny-Brown, D. and Russell, W. R. (1941). Experimental cerebral concussion. *Brain*, **64**, 93–164.
   This classical paper sorted out the gross mechanisms of various degrees of head injury. Worth reading because of its historical interest.
Foda, M. A. A. and Marmarou, A. (1994). A new model of diffuse brain injury in rats. Part II: Morphological characterisation. *Journal of Neurosurgery*, **80**, 301–13.
Gennarelli, T. A., Thibault, L. E., Adams, J. H., Graham, D. I., Thompson, C. J., and Marcincin, R. P. (1982). Diffuse axonal injury and traumatic coma in the primate. *Annals of Neurology*, **12**, 564–74.
   The definitive paper on primate injury, with experimental work unlikely to be repeated.
Gronwall, D. and Wrightson, P. (1980). Duration of post-traumatic amnesia after mild head injury. *Journal of Clinical Neuropsychology*, **2**, 51–60.
Hayes, R. H. and Dixon, C. E. (1994). Neurochemical changes in mild head injury. *Seminars in Neurology*, **14**, 25–31.
   A review by an authority in this field.
Jacobs, A., Put, E., Ingels, M., Put, T., and Bossuyt, A. (1996). One year follow-up of Technetium-99m-HPAO SPECT in mild head injury. *Journal of Nuclear Medicine*, **37**, 1605–9.
   A very well planned clinical and imaging study of perfusion in mild head injury.
Jünger, E. C., Newell, D. W., Grant, G. A., Avellino, A. M., Ghatan, S., Douville, C. M., *et al.* (1997). Cerebral autoregulation following minor head injury. *Journal of Neurosurgery*, **86**, 425–32.
Levin, H. S., Williams, D. H., Eisenberg, H. M., and High, W. M. (1992). Serial MRI and neurobehavioural findings after mild to moderate closed head injury. *Journal of Neurology, Neurosurgery and Psychiatry*, **55**, 255–62.

Oppenheimer, D. R. (1968). Microscopic lesions in the brain following head injury. *Journal of Neurology, Neurosurgery and Psychiatry,* **31**, 299–306.
The classical paper describing axonal rupture in mild injury in humans.

Povlishock, J. T. and Christman, C. W. (1995). Pathobiology of traumatically induced axonal injury in animals and humans: a review of current thoughts. *Journal of Neurotrauma,* **12**, 555–64.

Sakas, D. E. and Whitwell, H. L. (1997). Neurological episodes after minor head injury and trigeminovascular activation. *Medical Hypotheses,* **48**, 431–5.
Discusses the possible role of hyperperfusion in children's head injury and other situations.

Strich, S. J. (1961). Shearing of nerve fibres as a cause of brain damage due to head injury. *Lancet,* **2**, 443–8.

Wilson, J. T. L., Teasdale, G. M., Hadley, G. M., Wiedmann, K. D., and Lang, D. (1994). Post-traumatic amnesia: still a valuable yardstick. *Journal of Neurology, Neurosurgery and Psychiatry,* **57**, 198–201.

Yarnell, P. R. and Lynch, S. (1970). Retrograde memory immediately after concussion. *Lancet,* **i**, 863–4.

4
Management in the acute stage

Introduction

In Chapter 2 we offered a definition of mild head injury in the acute stage. It specified that there should have been an injury to the head with a disturbance of neurological function, that when first assessed there should be a GCS score of 13–15 which was steady or improving, and that there should be no focal neurological signs. In such a patient, after looking at any other injuries and at their general condition, the question of management will be decided largely on the possibility of complications, principally intracranial haemorrhage. Though this could be settled by continuing observations in the ED this is usually not practical and a system of assessment of risk is needed, which can contribute to the decision whether a patient can safely be discharged to home management or whether admission to hospital or transfer to higher level care is needed.

Assessment of this risk will be one of the major concerns of this chapter. We will first examine the factors associated with the development of complications, and then present a scheme for assessment in a form which may be useful as instructions for members of the staff of an ED. Lastly we will comment on the needs of patients with mild head injury who have been admitted to hospital either for observation of their neurological state or for treatment of other injuries. We will not comment on treatment at the scene of the accident, transport, or the general management of the patient in the ED; these are covered in texts on emergency medicine and usually determined by local conventions.

Risk factors in the development of acute complications

In patients with a GCS score of 13–15 when first seen, clinical signs of a risk of complications are the following.

(1) When the GCS score is initially 13–14, failure to improve over 4 h of observation, or with GCS 15, deterioration.

(2) A focal neurological deficit – motor, sensory, speech, balance.

(3) Persistent nausea, vomiting, or severe headache.

(4) Soft tissue injury or indications of skull fracture – bruising or full thickness wound of scalp or forehead, periorbital swelling, haemo-tympanum or mastoid bruising, or cerebrospinal fluid (CSF) from the nose or ear.

If any of these signs are present, further investigation is needed.

Further investigation

CT scans

In this context the primary function of a CT scan is to detect intracranial haemorrhage. There are several accounts of how often it is found in patients who fulfil the initial criteria of mild head injury. The figures vary considerably, depending on the stage at which the level of conscious-ness was assessed and the observer's experience, whether all patients had a CT scan or only those with suggestive clinical signs, and on the causes of injury most common in the reporting unit's catchment area.

For practical purposes data are needed which relate the risk of haem-orrhage to definite clinical signs; a good example of this is given by Dunham *et al.* (1996). They were concerned with the incidence of haemorrhage of any degree seen on CT scans, and found that major determinants were the age of the patient, the GCS score when seen at approximately one hour after the accident, and the presence of soft tissue injury to the scalp and upper facial area. Their figures for patients aged 14–60 are shown in Table 1; for those over 60 the incidence for a GCS score of 15 and no soft tissue injury was 5.8 per cent, and for others 16 per cent or greater. When there was a fracture of the vault the likeli-hood of haemorrhage was increased 15 times, and of the base of the skull by 30 times.

Table 1   Incidence of intracranial haemorrhage seen in CT scan, ages 14–60

	GCS 15	GCS 14	GCS 13
No soft tissue injury (%)	1.5	7.1	16.1
Soft tissue injury (%)	6.2	19.9	35.2
Number of cases	1481	435	116

Source: Dunham *et al.* 1996.

Though intracranial haemorrhage of some degree was seen in these patients, only a small proportion of them needed a craniotomy – 2.3 per cent when there was no soft tissue injury, and 8.2 per cent when this was present. Seventy-five per cent of the craniotomies were due to deterioration occurring within 4 h of arrival at the ED.

Skull radiography

A skull fracture indicates that there has been an impact of some severity, and its presence makes intracranial haemorrhage and infective complications more likely. In the past, skull radiographs played an important part in management of mild head injury, though when they were used as a routine on all cases the return was small. Now where CT scans are readily available, when a fracture is suspected a scan will usually be done in preference because of its ability to detect intracranial haemorrhage. Skull radiographs may, however, be used when there is a full thickness scalp wound and no other indication for CT. Again, when CT is not available, skull films may help in the decision whether to transfer the patient to a higher level centre.

Comment on management policies

Given that a guiding consideration is the avoidance of major complications, should it be policy that a CT scan should be obtained routinely on all head injury patients?

We have seen that there is sound evidence that careful clinical assessment and the facility to observe patients for four or five hours will select a group in which complications are very unlikely. In the rest of the patients a CT scan will be needed, and this will determine whether further observation is needed or intervention is likely. There are therefore good clinical grounds for a discretionary policy.

Other considerations can be important. An increasingly litigious society may demand that every possible investigation should be done, even if there is no good clinical indication, so that if there has been no CT scan and there is a complication the doctor and their organization may be sued.

There is also the question of cost. Though the uncertainty in a borderline case of mild head injury can be dispelled by a CT, observing the patient for a longer period in the ED or in a hospital bed is also effective. Whether it is cheaper to obtain a CT will depend on local circumstances. It would be very difficult for a smaller hospital if a CT became required practice and all mild head injuries had to be transferred to a larger centre.

In the scheme that follows it will be taken that a discretionary policy is in place; if local conditions make it desirable that all patients have a CT scan the necessary changes will be evident.

Principles of management of less severe head injuries in emergency departments

The problems

The treatment of the more severe injuries is taken over by specialist teams. The remainder, in general patients with a GCS score of 13–15 when first seen, are likely to recover with supportive treatment only and are the responsibility of emergency department staff. The decisions that they have to make are the following.

(1) At the initial assessment, what is the risk of complications?

(2) Does the risk of intracranial haemorrhage make a CT scan neces-sary? Should the skull be X-rayed?

(3) If there is no immediate indication of a complication, for how long should the patient be observed?

(4) After this period of observation, should they be allowed to go home or should they be admitted to hospital for further observation?

(5) How and when should scalp wounds be treated?

(6) What follow-up should be arranged?

The factors

(1) The risk of rapid onset/low incidence/high mortality complications – principally intracranial haemorrhage.

(2) The risk of infective complications – nose/ear fractures with CSF leak, unsuspected penetrating injuries.

(3) The likely symptoms in the next 24 h.

(4) Other injuries.

(5) The patient's age, general condition, and pre-existing problems.

(6) The care available to the patient out of hospital.

Patients who are at risk of intracranial haemorrhage

(1) Patients with a GCS score of <13 on arrival and patients in whom the GCS deteriorates during observation need to have intracranial haemorrhage excluded.

(2) The risk remains significant when the GCS score is at first 13 or 14 and then does not improve over a period of observation of up to 4 h. The risk is minimal when the GCS score has been steady at 15 for a similar period.

(3) Patients with focal neurological abnormalities.

(4) Patients with definite soft tissue injuries of the upper face, forehead, and scalp, in whom intracranial haemorrhage is 2–3 times more likely.

(5) Patients aged 60 and over, who are 2–3 times more likely to have an intracranial haemorrhage.

Patients who are at risk of infective complications

(1) Frontal bruising, periorbital bruising, or damage to the nose, or mastoid bruising or haemotympanum, indicate a risk of infection entering the subarachnoid space.

(2) Scalp lacerations may overlie open fractures; particularly in small children a penetrating injury of the brain may lie under a small cut.

Indications for CT scan

(1) Patients with a GCS score of 15 on arrival and no more than minor soft tissue injury should be observed, with a scan only if they deteriorate.

(2) Patients with a GCS score of 13–14 on arrival but no soft tissue injury may be observed for 2–3 h. If the GCS rises to 15 and there is no deterioration, observation may continue.

(3) Patients with a GCS score of 13–15 who have significant soft tissue injuries should have a CT scan.

(4) Patients with a focal neurological abnormality should have a CT scan.

Management after initial assessment

(1) Patients who have not needed a scan, or who have had a scan which has shown no abnormality should be observed for a minimum period of 4 h and then if neurologically normal may be considered for discharge. If they are not neurologically normal, observation should be continued; whether in the ED or admitted to hospital being a matter for administrative decision.

(2) Patients who have had a scan which has shown intracranial haemorrhage should be admitted to hospital for observation. In most cases the haemorrhage is minor, will not require operation, and will allow

discharge after a few days. However, these patients form a group in which there is a greater probability of persistent problems.

Determination of neurological normality

(1) Glasgow Coma Scale score should be 15, and the patient should be alert and orientated with normal recent memory. Orientation should be tested by a standard series of questions (see Appendix 1). Recent memory should be tested by the ability to recall test statements after a 15 minute interval. Note that orientation and memory are independent functions and that each should be normal.

(2) Vision, eye movements, pupil reactions, hearing, gait, and balance should all be normal.

(3) Headache should be mild and tolerable. There should be no nausea, and they should not have vomited in the last 2 h.

(4) Cardiovascular signs of increasing intracranial pressure would not be expected in patients normal to the preceding tests. Nevertheless, pulse, blood pressure, and respiratory rate should be noted and any deviation from normal explained.

Management if a CT scan is not easily available

(1) Patients in whom a CT scan would not have been recommended (Indications for CT scan, items (1) and (2) above) are managed in the same way.

(2) Patients with marked soft tissue injuries should have a skull X-ray. Those neurologically normal and without a fracture can be considered for discharge. Those with a fracture and/or not neurologically normal should be admitted for observation.

(3) Patients aged 60+ should be admitted for observation, unless the injury is trivial.

(4) Patients showing neurological deterioration will need transfer to higher level care.

Scalp lacerations

(1) The risks of a scalp laceration are infection when foreign bodies are retained and the compounding of a skull fracture. A low incidence/high risk situation is a perforating wound driving bone and dirt through the dura. In one series a quarter of cerebral abscesses seen were due to neglected scalp lacerations.

(2) All scalp lacerations should therefore be inspected carefully, the hair shaved well away from the wound, and the skin cleaned. If the

laceration does not go through the aponeurotic layer it can be sutured. If the aponeurotic layer has been divided and if periosteum is visible, the wound should be explored carefully for foreign bodies or other soiling, cleaned and sutured. An X-ray should then be done to see if there is a fracture or if any foreign bodies have been missed in the exploration.

Children – important differences

(1) Children under seven respond to trauma in a way which differs from that seen in the adult, because of the size of the head and the relative weakness of the neck muscles and because the brain is incompletely myelinated and responds in a different way to the forces of acceleration.

(2) The child's skull is more elastic than the adult's and as the dura mater is firmly adherent to it, the meningeal arteries may be torn without there being a fracture. Extradural haemorrhage can occur without a loss of consciousness, bruise, or fracture.

(3) In children in their first five years the initial response to injury may be slight, with either a short period of unconsciousness or none at all, but drowsiness, nausea, and vomiting may come on up to three or four hours later.

(4) Assessment of a child's neurological state is difficult because of
   (i)   problems of estimating higher cerebral function (a Glasgow Coma Scale modified for children is given in Appendix 7);
   (ii) the emotional response to trauma;
   (iii) confusion of natural tiredness with pathological drowsiness.

(5) After initial assessment a child with a GCS score of 15, no neurological abnormalities, and no or minimal soft tissue damage, should be observed for at least 4 h; if there is no deterioration they may be discharged to the care of their parents.

   Children with an initial GCS score of 13 or 14 and no other abnormalities may be observed for an hour or two and if they recover to a GCS score of 15 and are otherwise normal they may be candidates for discharge after a further 4 h.

   Children with marked soft tissue damage, neurological abnormalities, or a GCS score which fails to improve or deteriorates are at risk from intracranial haemorrhage and a CT scan should be done. If this is not available, transfer to a higher level service should be considered.

(6) When a CT scan has been indicated and has been normal the child should be kept under observation. There may be reluctance to admit a child to hospital. The hard facts are that deterioration can still occur,

possibly with seizures, and that proper observation of a small child is difficult enough for professionals and impossible for parents. Hospitals should be able to make admission more acceptable by accommodating a parent with the child.

(7) The same considerations about X-rays and lacerations apply to children as to adults. Note particularly the ease with which a sharp projection – the axle of a toy or a nail – can perforate the skull and dura through a 2 mm laceration.

(8) Note particularly an important and potentially fatal complication of head injury in young children – status epilepticus. Rapid and effective control is needed.

Older people

Older people, those over the age of 60, are more likely to develop intracranial haemorrhage. As well as having more fragile vessels they may be taking aspirin or NSAIDs which increase the risk of bleeding. A CT is therefore indicated in almost every case, unless the injury was minimal, the GCS score on arrival was 15, and there was no soft tissue injury. Because of the risks it is wise to admit patients of this age to hospital, even if only for 24 h. Many have significant medical problems, principally cardiac and respiratory disease, which may be made worse by the accident. They may live alone or have only other old people to look after them; the injury may be the event which puts an end to independent living. Before discharge they should therefore be assessed by a medical social worker and possibly seen by a geriatrician.

Ethanol and other drugs

As many as 40 per cent of patients who come to EDs with a mild head injury have been taking alcohol and an uncertain proportion other drugs which could affect their level of consciousness. The circumstances of the accident and the smell will suggest that ethanol is a factor. Blood levels or breath tests may indicate how relevant it is – confusion should not be attributed to ethanol unless the blood level is greater than 50 mmol/l (0.2 g/dl) and coma unless the level is greater than 75 mmol/l (0.3 g/dl). Other drugs, alone or with ethanol, may be suspected and evidence of this may come from companions or needle marks.

Younger patients who appear to be intoxicated, with a GCS score of 13–14 and no marked soft tissue injury, maybe observed for 2 h or so and if their conscious level improves significantly further observation and disposal as for other patients is reasonable. In older patients with a GCS score of 13–14 the chance of complications is greater, a period of observation carries risks, and an early CT is advisable. When the head injury appears to be playing a minor part, the protocol for possible drug overdosage should be started.

Advice and follow-up for patients discharged home

1. The patient and those who will look after them must be impressed with the need to report at once if there is any deterioration in the level of consciousness, limb weakness, or leakage of fluid from the nose or ear. Patients and relatives are often not receptive when they leave the emergency department and it is helpful for them to have a handout describing the immediate dangers and possible later symptoms. It is prudent that they should sign in the clinical notes that this has been received.

2. Patients and relatives should be told about the symptoms they can expect, when they should return to work, drive a car, or play sport. Useful guidelines are as follows.

*   *Return to work.* Fifty per cent of people will feel unduly tired and have difficulty in concentrating for 10–14 days after concussion. They may be able to cope with work, but at a lower level of efficiency, and it is best to start part time if they can. Most young people should be working full time after 14 days; older people will usually take longer.

*   *Driving.* It is unsafe to drive for at least 24 h after the accident. Reactions are likely to be slow for several more days and driving should not be allowed until the patient is quite free of symptoms. Then they may start with caution, avoiding heavy traffic or long trips.

*   *Sport.* Ordinary exercise can start when tiredness and dizziness allow. Contact sports where concussion is a risk should not be played for at least three weeks.

3. Patients should be told that if they do not feel back to normal again by 14 days after the injury they should seek advice, either from their own doctor or from a source nominated by the emergency department.

4. An example of a simple information sheet is given in Appendix 2. This is suitable to give to patients aged up to the mid 40s who have been allowed home after observation in the ED. In older patients, or those with special risks, it will be worth while giving them more explicit information about possible longer term effects, and an example of a pamphlet designed to do this is in Appendix 4. Most patients find this helpful.

Patients with a mild head injury who have been admitted to hospital

Patients with a mild head injury who have been admitted to hospital will fall into two groups. Some will have been assessed in the ED and either did not recover quickly or had signs indicating the possibility of complications. Others will have been admitted because of limb or trunk trauma but had an incidental mild head injury.

Most of those admitted primarily because of their head injury will be observed for 24–48 h and will then be fit to return home. Some, including those who had a CT scan which showed minor intracranial haemorrhage, will recover more slowly, but without the obvious complications that would put them into the category of a major injury. Because these patients have been more severely affected than those sent home from the ED, they are more likely to experience problems during recovery. It is important that they and their family should be aware of this, and are told how to get help. The information sheets given in Appendices 2 and 4 should be useful. Particular care should be taken with those at special risk, people whose work depends on concentration and memory, and in particular students and professional people.

When patients have been admitted with limb or trunk trauma a mild head injury may be neglected while more serious injuries are being treated. This is of little importance in the acute stage, but problems with behaviour and cognition may remain when the patient has recovered from the other injuries. If this is not recognized they may be encouraged to return to work before they have fully recovered from their head injury. The result may not only be personal problems but a damaging reaction from their employer.

It is important that at the time patients leave hospital these issues are discussed with the patient and their relatives and that arrangements are made to follow them up, either at a hospital clinic or by their general practitioner. If symptoms persist, they may need formal neurological and neuropsychological assessment.

Patients seen by their general practitioner

Many patients with milder head injuries will consult their general practitioner rather than go to hospital, often a day or more after the accident when they find that the headache has not gone away or when they have other symptoms such as dizziness or visual problems. The same principles of management will apply. A proportion of the patients will also encounter persisting symptoms (see Chapter 2) and referral for specialist assessment will be needed.

References and Further Reading

Dunham, C. M., Coates, S., and Cooper, C. (1996). Compelling evidence for discretionary brain computed tomographic imaging in those patients with mild

cognitive impairment after blunt trauma. *Journal of Trauma, Infection and Critical Care,* **41**, 679–86.
This provides an excellent statistical basis for the management of milder head injury in the ED.
Roy, C. W., Pentland, B., and Miller, J. D. (1986). The causes and consequences of minor head injury in the elderly. *Injury,* **17**, 220–3.
This gives an account of the complicating factors in head injury in the elderly.
Rutherford, W. H. (ed.) (1989). *Accident and emergency medicine.* Churchill Livingstone, Edinburgh.

5

Clinical picture after mild head injury

Introduction

Most people who have had a mild head injury experience unpleasant symptoms for a few days, usually of headache, lethargy, and irritability, but will be back to their normal activities in two or three weeks. In some these symptoms fail to resolve. Their headache continues and their sight and balance may be disturbed. They have difficulty with concentration and memory which prevents their returning to work, and there may be changes in their behaviour and personality. Lastly there is a small group of patients who have had less marked but still disabling symptoms for months or years before it is realized or accepted that they have been caused by a head injury.

The symptoms in these patients can be considered in four main categories – somatic, cognitive, behavioural, and stress related. The mixture varies from patient to patient and there are different patterns depending on factors such as the time after injury, age, occupation, and personality. Always a major component is the reaction of the patient to the symptoms and the disability they cause, and this stress results in a variety of secondary problems.

We will describe the patient's condition in the days immediately after the injury, the recovery in the usual case, and then when symptoms persist. The picture will be that which can be gathered from talking to the patient and their relatives. We will then discuss some points in the history taking and clinical diagnosis. The medical investigation of somatic features and the neuropsychological assessment will be dealt with in later chapters, as will the special features in older people, in children, and after sports injuries.

The clinical picture

The usual recovery from mild head injury

The patient will either have been observed in hospital for one or two days, or have been allowed to go home after being assessed in a hospital emergency department or by a general practitioner. There can be a range of symptoms. Some will have minor discomfort due to bruising or neck strain and little else. Others will experience more severe symptoms for a number of days, most often headache, nausea, photophobia, blurred vision, and drowsiness.

These somatic symptoms will usually have cleared after ten days or so, but the patient's attempt to get back to normal life may be obstructed by difficulty in settling down to a task, inability to read for more than a few minutes, absent mindedness, and irritability. Concentration will often bring on headache and exercise may make it worse. Again in most people these symptoms will settle within a further week or two and it will become practical for them to get back to normal activity and work. It is, however, likely to be several weeks more before they feel entirely recovered.

To look at the recovery from mild head injury when complicating factors such as compensation and employment would have least effect the authors looked at the recovery of a group of fit young men in regular employment who had been concussed, seen in an emergency department, and then allowed home after a period of observation (Wrightson and Gronwall 1981). Eighty per cent of them were back at work within a week, 90 per cent after two weeks, and all within a month. However, though they were back at work, at first around a half felt strange – detached, not 'a hundred per cent' – and thought that they were not doing their work as well as usual. At the same time their leisure activities were disturbed, they couldn't be bothered to play sport or go out in the evening, and they went to bed one or two hours earlier than usual. Almost all had returned to normal by a month, but several continued to have symptoms for up to three months and one or two said they could still notice an effect after two years, mostly problems with memory and concentration.

Impaired recovery – when patients come for help

Though most people recover completely from a mild head injury within a month or two, in a small proportion symptoms are either present in a more severe form to begin with or continue without getting better. Based on the time that they ask for help, people who come with these symptoms fall into three groups.

The early group

These are patients who still have the symptoms that were present in the early days after the injury. Their condition may have continued unchanged or the symptoms may have cleared to some extent and then returned when the patient tried to get back to normal activity. Headache, dizziness, forgetfulness, irritability, and fatigue are prominent and there are often indications of stress, especially a change of sleep pattern to waking in the small hours.

The middle group

These patients come for help one to several months after the injury. There is often a history of symptoms of the early group, but these may not have been severe and the patient may have put up with them, perhaps under medical supervision, expecting a recovery which did not occur. Usually the main complaints are of poor memory and concentration, and usually these can be confirmed by an appropriate neuropsychological assessment. Fatigue, irritability, and symptoms of stress are usually present and headache, dizziness, and other somatic symptoms are frequent. The symptoms may not have resulted in a serious limitation until the patient tried to return to normal activity.

The late group

In this group there is a yet smaller number of people who have been living at a disadvantage for months or years after a mild head injury. They may have just been able to get by at daily activities, at home or at work, but have lost their edge and their enjoyment of life. The problem has often been a cognitive one, with poor memory and concentration and abnormal fatigue, and perhaps impaired insight or self-control. Somatic symptoms may be present but are seen less often, perhaps because they encourage an earlier diagnosis. Often the patient has adapted and continued for a long period unchanged until some extra stress, perhaps at work or in the family, proves too much for them to cope with and they break down. When they eventually seek advice a diagnosis of depression is often made. The connection with injury may not seem definite, and if it is proposed may be disputed by insurers.

The symptoms when recovery is delayed

The pattern of symptoms when recovery is delayed is as consistent as any in clinical medicine. In some it is seen for only a week or two, in others it continues with only slow changes for months or years, and in a few it becomes permanent.

Here we will deal with the general cognitive and behavioural aspects of the picture, describing the symptoms as the patient relates them. In later chapters we will examine their neurological and neuropsychological basis.

Forgetfulness

This is perhaps the commonest complaint. Patients forget trivial affairs, where they put their spectacles, that there is a kettle on the stove, why they went upstairs. They read but forget what was on the previous page, take messages and then forget to relay them. In contrast recall of important events before the accident and of basic information and learned skills is mostly unaffected.

Concentration

Patients find it is difficult to keep their mind on what they are doing. The slightest distraction such as a radio playing in the background will spoil their concentration. Even more difficult is a task which needs attention to more than one input. They can cope with talking to one person, but if they join a conversation with several people the thread is lost. Following a discussion round the table at a business meeting is impossible. Attention may lapse when they are travelling; they may reach their destination but not know how they got there, or suddenly realize they are lost. They may finish working on a familiar task and find they have missed an essential step.

Thinking

There is a general fall-off of mental energy and capacity. They are uninterested in reading (apart from forgetting what they have read). It is difficult to sort out their thoughts and express them, particularly when integrative or abstract thinking is needed. Conversation tends to be roundabout and diffuse.

Fatigue

Abnormal tiredness probably has a more direct effect on a patient's life than any other factor, partly because in itself it limits performance and partly because it increases the effect of the other symptoms, creating a vicious cycle.

In most cases the fatigue is brought on most quickly by cognitive effort, desk work, reading, or any activity that needs attention. Physical effort does have some effect, particularly in the early stages when it may bring on somatic symptoms, but later it is better tolerated.

Characteristically, providing their sleep has not been disturbed, the patient starts the day with some feeling of energy. Then, fairly suddenly, often they say like a curtain coming down, they find they are struggling to keep going and can't make sense of what they're doing. Frequently at this point they begin to experience a headache. If they recognize this warning and rest for an hour or two they may recover and be able to start again for another period. If they neglect the warning and go on working until they can cope no longer they bring on a state of severe fatigue which will stop them doing anything productive for the rest of the day; often it will persist and prevent useful work the next day, or even for longer.

Comments by the family or pressure at work can make the situation worse. It is difficult for others to understand the limitations imposed by the fatigue and they can encourage or embarrass the patient into continuing in spite of it. When a patient who has been improving starts to regress, this sort of situation will often be uncovered.

Lack of insight

Patients may be unable to appreciate their own actions and realize when they may be harmful to themselves or objectionable to others.

In the first days after a mild head injury a few patients will act uncharacteristically, denying that they have problems and insisting on returning to their usual activities, including dangerous areas such as driving. Later it may be difficult to persuade them that they are not ready for work, or that they should start part-time. Usually after a week or two they realize, often quite suddenly, what they have been doing, and often find it difficult to believe they could have been so unwise.

In some patients the lack of insight continues. It may take the form of denial that there are problems, either at work or in the family or social area. In others there is a more subtle and distressing loss of the normal social restraints with inappropriate behaviour. Extremes of this sort are rare after a mild injury, but a few of the more severely injured patients do become overfamiliar, do not respect personal space, or may make sly sexual overtures.

Irritability

Irritability, impatience, and poor self-control are common symptoms and affect all areas of everyday life.

In the early stages it is the patient's family that is most affected. Minor domestic irritations provoke an exaggerated response and children's games and noises are not tolerated. Later, at the stage of return to work, irritability may be a major problem, and the minor hassles of business can provoke an explosive response which can have disastrous results.

Sensitivity to light and noise

Patients are commonly sensitive to light and need to wear dark glasses, sometimes even indoors; this problem sometimes remains when most of the other symptoms have cleared.

Sensitivity to noise has two aspects. When people are functioning normally they can disregard irrelevant sound such as other people talking or background music, but when concentration is impaired the unwanted input cannot be shut out. The other aspect is that, as with light, sound of any sort can be an irritant. Children playing or pop music are typical sources of irritation in the early stages and often create family problems; later intolerance of noise on the factory floor may be a major factor in making it difficult to get back to work.

Loss of libido and sexual activity

As patients recover and begin to expect a more normal way of life they often find they have little or no sexual urge. In some this continues longer than most of the other symptoms and is a major factor in preventing a return to a full and normal life.

Anxiety and depression

Anxiety is an important component in the reaction to any illness, and if it is unrelieved may delay recovery or lead to clinical depression.

In the first week or two after a mild injury headaches, dizziness, and other somatic symptoms will be of most concern to the patient. When they are seen at this stage they may be anxious but reasonably confident about the outcome, much as they would in any other illness of comparable impact. As the somatic symptoms become less intense they may become aware that they can't remember things or concentrate properly. This can be very frightening, and talking about it later when the cause has been explained a patient will often say that they thought that they were going mad, and what a relief it was to know that there was a physical explanation.

When the patient has passed through the earlier stages of recovery and has accepted that there are cognitive and other symptoms, but is finding that they are not clearing as they had hoped, they are likely to become stressed and perhaps depressed. Often the first indication that this has happened is a change in sleep pattern. In the earlier stages most patients will need to go to bed early, get up late, and sleep deeply between. As they become anxious they will wake after two or three hours of sleep, remain awake and worrying for a further period, and then drift off to sleep again, eventually waking to feel tired and unrefreshed. It is important to recognize this pattern, for the management of anxiety and fatigue may be the most important task at this stage.

If progress is slow, as disability persists and the prospect of a return to a previous lifestyle becomes remote, there may be a more severe reaction and patients may become clinically depressed, with hopelessness, apathy, and a loss of will to continue with rehabilitation; in a few cases this will lead to suicide. People with a previous history of depression will be more likely to enter this state and will need more than the usual amount of support.

The effect on the family

The clinical assessment of mild head injury is incomplete without considering the effect that it has on the partner and family, for this will in turn reflect on the patient.

The first reaction will be relief that the injury was mild, and in the majority of cases this relief is justified by a rapid improvement and return to normal family relations and activity in a few weeks.

When recovery is prolonged a variety of reactions develop. There is anxiety about the true nature of the condition, whether there has been more than a simple head injury, and if there should be more tests. They may wonder if the doctors they have seen are sufficiently competent, and ask for a second opinion. Sometimes the patient feels that they are going mad, and the family may feel this too. The question then may come up whether all these symptoms are in fact real or if they are putting it on for money or sympathy or just laziness – this can be a concern to the family as well as to outsiders. Adding to these anxieties it is likely that there are financial burdens, especially if the patient is the major income earner.

Lastly, and perhaps the most difficult of all, there is the burden of having to live with the patient's symptoms. Forgetfulness and disorganization are annoying. Irritability is a major problem and will be provoked by much of the business of running a home and looking after children. Social life may come to a stop and the loss of libido may be hard to hear.

Somatic symptoms

These will be discussed in the next chapter.

Practical considerations in history taking

It is important for immediate and later use that a full history should be available. This is best obtained in the first place with the least amount of prompting. A pro forma or checklist may be used, but with caution as it may generate a rigidity of approach. It may be of most use for recording progress, particularly if there is provision for grading the severity of individual symptoms. A useful and well tried system is the Rivermead post-concussion symptoms (PCS) questionnaire, which is included in Appendix 6.

Care should be taken to include a full account of the accident, both to match it with the clinical features and for possible later use in litigation.

The duration of coma and the GCS when first seen, together with retrograde and post-traumatic amnesia should be stated clearly.

There should be a general medical history, with details of any previous head injuries.

To obtain a more objective account of the patient's symptoms and condition it is important to talk to the patient's partner and family. At this time or later it will be necessary to get details of the patient's education and present and past employment. This will help in assessing their current state and in advising on preparation for return to work, and possibly in litigation.

When the history has been completed in this way the next step is a general medical and neurological examination and a neuropsychological assessment. These are described in the following chapters.

Comment on the clinical picture

In a typical case the history of injury and the subsequent symptoms will usually leave the diagnosis in little doubt. Marked somatic symptoms may suggest the possibility of a gross structural basis for them, such as a subdural haematoma, and further investigation may be needed to rule this out. Formal neuropsychological testing will confirm the diagnosis, quantify the general depression of cognitive function, and show up any areas where there is a particularly marked deficit which may need special attention in management.

There may, however, be uncertainty when there is an excessive or atypical reaction to the injury, which suggests either pre-existing emotional instability or deliberate exaggeration. The doubt can usually be resolved by the neuropsychological assessment, which will show a disproportion between the deficits and the symptoms. Obvious inconsistencies within the tests can suggest frank malingering.

The greatest difficulty in diagnosis is experienced with patients with symptoms of the late group. The connection with injury may be uncertain. The emotional reaction to a long lasting unexplained disability may suggest that the symptoms were of psychiatric origin from the outset. If there is negotiation for compensation it may appear that the symptoms are being exaggerated. In coming to a decision, most weight will again be placed on the result of neuropsychological testing. A clear deficit in one or more cognitive functions will support an organic origin. Also very important is well documented evidence of a change in capacity at work or in home-making clearly related to the time of an accident. When the problem is predominantly one of family and social relations, or of fatigue alone, and the neuropsychological findings are equivocal, diagnosis may depend on the consistency of the history, and be difficult to appreciate by someone not familiar with the syndrome.

Further reading

Alexander, M. P. (1995). Mild traumatic brain injury: pathophysiology, natural history, and clinical management. *Neurology,* **45**, 1253–60.
This paper provides a useful discussion of these clinical features.
Rimel, R. W., Giordani, B., Barth, J. T., Boll, T. J., and Jane, D. A. (1981). Disability caused by minor head injury. *Neurosurgery,* **9**, 221–5.
The paper by the authors was an attempt to see what symptoms occurred after minimal injury in a group of young men who were at the time of injury in employment and returned to work within a month. The papers by Rimel *et al.* and by Rutherford *et al.* report the symptoms of groups of unselected consecutive patients with minor head injuries admitted to hospital; the incidence of secondary symptoms is consequently higher than in the first study.
Rutherford, W. H., Merrett, J. D., and McDonald, J. R. (1977). Sequelae of concussion caused by minor head injuries. *Lancet,* **1**, 1–4.
Rutherford, W. H., Merrett, J. D., and McDonald, J. R. (1978). Symptoms at one year following concussion from minor head injuries. *Injury,* **10**, 225–30.
Wrightson, P. and Gronwall, D. (1981). Time off work and symptoms after minor head injury. *Injury,* **12**, 445–54.

6
Neurological assessment

Introduction

In a previous chapter we discussed the cognitive and behavioural symptoms seen when recovery from mild head injury is delayed or incomplete. here we will deal with the somatic symptoms, describing the clinical features, the examination, concepts of mechanism, and specific treatment. Some of the conditions can be managed by the generalist to whom this book is addressed, others will need to be referred to specialists.

HEADACHE

Introduction

Headache is the commonest symptom recorded in most studies of mild head injury. Most patients expect to have a headache in the first few days after injury. When symptoms persist or recur later it may be more natural to complain of headache than of the more subtle problems of memory and concentration or of anxiety and depression. Often therefore it is the first symptom mentioned, though others may be more disabling. It is nevertheless a symptom which means a great deal to the patient and needs to be managed efficiently and with respect.

Because there are no objective signs or measures of the severity of the headache and because the cause may be difficult to define, headache is often taken either to be secondary to anxiety and depression, or to be exaggerated. Certainly anxiety and headache are interdependent, one fuelling the other, and it may be difficult to say which comes first. As well, the prominence of headache in some claims for compensation has suggested that it is simulated, though numerous studies have shown that it usually persists after the claim has been settled.

With this in mind, it is necessary to be particularly thorough in the diagnosis of the causes of headache.

Investigation

A detailed history is needed. Where is the pain felt? is it sharp, an ache, or throbbing? Is it always the same sort of headache, or different at different times? Is it getting better with time, or worse? Is it accompanied by visual symptoms or nausea? Does it come on at any particular time of day? Does anything in particular bring it on? How long does it last for? Is there anything – rest, medicine – that makes it better? Worse? What do you do when it comes on – rest, go to bed, carry on in spite of it? Did you have headaches before the accident, and were they like these? Were they diagnosed as migraine? Does anyone in your family have migraine?

A thorough examination of the cranial nerves is needed. Are there areas of tenderness or hyperaesthesia in the scalp or neck? Is the range of movement of the cervical spine limited or painful? Is there muscle tenderness, or are there trigger points in the cervical muscles? Tenderness over the greater occipital nerves? Soreness on pressure over the front or maxillary sinuses? Loss of infraorbital nerve sensation?

Varieties of headache

Early headache

This occurs in the first few days after the injury. It is usually felt all over the head, but worse where there is a bruise. It is often throbbing and may be accompanied by nausea and is usually made worse by coughing or moving around. There is sensitivity to light. The neck is often stiff, with pain on movement and muscle tenderness (major damage such as injury to the cervical spine will have been excluded in the initial assessment).

The symptoms are usually self-limiting. The headache can be helped, though usually not dispelled completely, by analgesics such as paracetamol, codeine compounds, or NSAIDs. When headache of this sort is severe and persistent in the early days after injury it may be due to a subacute extradural or subdural haematoma; care must be taken not to obscure warning signs with stronger analgesia.

Headache of increased intracranial pressure

When more severe headache continues for more than a week or two after injury a chronic subdural haematoma or post-traumatic hydrocephalus may be suggested. When these conditions are present the headache is usually persistent, present first thing in the morning, and worse with coughing or straining. The pain is generally felt all over the head, but may be worse on the side of a haematoma. As symptoms progress there may be nausea or vomiting. On examination there may be papilloedema or localizing signs but often there is only the headache to suggest the pathology.

Continuing headache in the first month or two after a mild injury is a common reason for referral for a further opinion. A CT scan has to be done, because of the serious possibilities, but in fact structural pathology is not often found; further diagnosis and management can then go on.

Fatigue-related headache

This headache occurs typically in people with cognitive impairment and follows activity which requires concentration. It is usually felt all over the head, sometimes described as a tight band, and tends not to be throbbing. Often the patient is free from headache when they wake and in the first hour or two of the day, but the headache then comes on after a period when they have been trying to work or concentrate. The time free of headache is much the same from day to day, but is reduced when the work is more stressful. Physical activity, when there is no stress associated, does not typically produce this sort of headache. There may be cervical pain in association with the headache, due to muscle tension.

Rest, with a sleep if practical, gives the best relief. Analgesics have little effect. Care should be taken with their use, for it is one of the situations where patients may first use over-the-counter drugs to excess and then later develop drug-withdrawal headache. Management is that of the PCS as a whole, and essentially consists of adjusting the patient's activity to their capacity and dealing with any of the sources of additional stress.

Headache related to physical activity

More often in the early period after the injury patients may develop a headache, usually described as throbbing or pounding, when they exert themselves, either with hurrying, physical work, or exercise. The headache is usually general or frontal. There are no specific findings on examination.

For a period the patient should avoid the activity that provokes the headache and then start again gently and work up their tolerance. If the headache is severe or continues with mild activity a structural lesion may need to be excluded with a CT scan.

Referred musculoskeletal pain

This pain is felt most often in the occipital region and upper cervical muscles, and may radiate forward into the temporal areas. Usually it is steady and does not throb. It may interfere with sleep and is generally worse on getting up in the morning; it may then clear for a while and come back later in the day as the patient gets tired.

On examination there is likely to be some painful limitation of neck movement and there will be points of tenderness in the cervical muscles and occipital scalp, and over the greater occipital nerves. When the physical signs are marked, radiographs should be checked to be sure that there are no unnoticed bone lesions.

Treatment should begin with long acting NSAIDs at night and physio-therapy; tricyclic antidepressants may be useful if pain continues in spite of treatment. More severe or persistent pain may need referral to ortho-paedic or physical medicine specialists.

This variety of headache is often present at the same time as fatigue-related headache. One accentuates the other, and the combination is particularly hard for the patient to bear.

Migraine-like headache

Some patients have episodes of severe headache with nausea, vomiting, and photophobia and sometimes visual disturbances. Three types of such migraine-like headache can be recognized after head injury.

(1) Some patients who have suffered from migraine before the accident will experience one or more attacks in the period immediately after the injury, or attacks may occur more often than usual in the follow-ing months. These headaches will usually be recognized for what they are and be treated in the patient's customary way.

(2) Others who have not had migraine before will, within a few hours to a few weeks of the injury, start to have typical attacks of migraine. These should be managed in the same way as idiopathic migraine, in the first place with oral NSAIDs and an antiemetic, taken as soon as the typical symptoms are recognized. If after a proper trial this is ineffective, the headache is severe, and relief is needed, sumatriptan may be used. If the attacks are frequent prophylaxis with a β-blocker or amitriptyline may be worth while.

(3) 'Footballer's migraine'. Uncommonly an attack of typical migraine, with visual symptoms and nausea, can occur immediately after head-ing the ball, and at no other time. It appears to occur more often when the player has not been ready, and has not tightened his neck muscles to prevent his head moving with the impact. It can occur after any sort of closed head injury, but is only likely to be recognized when there are repeated events such as in boxing or sports. Some-times there is a period of confusion or visual blunting at the onset of the attack and then the condition may be confused with concus-sion. However, the symptoms can be expected to clear within 24 h

and neuropsychological testing will not show the changes seen after concussion. It is sensible to avoid the provocation, but if the player insists on continuing, it has been suggested that they take a dose either of ergotamine or an NSAID before the match.

'Cluster' type headache

The symptoms here are similar to those of the 'migrainous neuralgia' or 'cluster' headache. They tend to occur regularly for a week or two separated by longer intervals of freedom, though not at a specific time of day like the typical cluster headache. Whether it is a specific condition or a migraine variation is uncertain.

Unlike most other post-traumatic headaches the onset is spontaneous and not usually related to activity or fatigue. The pain is localized to one side of the head, usually to one temple or behind one eye; often there has been an injury in this area. There may be nausea and vomiting, and sometimes increased sensitivity to light, less commonly conjunctival injection, oedema around the eye, lacrimation and rhinorrhoea, or a Horner's syndrome. The pain is usually severe but lasts for a limited time, of the order of a few minutes to an hour.

In the attack an NSAID suppository may be tried, but may not work before the pain ceases spontaneously. Relief can sometimes be obtained by inhaling a high concentration of oxygen, with an effect after 10 minutes or so. If this is not practical or does not work, sumatriptan by injection is usually very effective. If the attacks are frequent, amitriptyline in small doses can be a useful prophylactic.

Persistent local pain

Pain at the site of an injury such as a scalp bruise is common in the early stages. It usually clears spontaneously but it may persist. When it does, it is often due to a localized high-energy impact such as being struck by a golf ball. The pain is usually felt over a limited area. It usually comes on spontaneously, though the area may be sensitive to touch or cold. There may be partial or complete loss of touch over the area as well as hypersensitivity, suggesting nerve damage at the point of impact. Occasionally the pain may seem to be related to an artery, and compression of the superficial temporal artery over the zygoma may relieve it. Management is often difficult. NSAIDs should be tried. Infiltration of the area with local anaesthetic may help, and transcutaneous electrical nerve stimulation (TENS) can be tried. If the severity of the pain justifies its use, carbamazepine may be effective. Sometimes none of these measures succeed, and more general pain management may be called for as described below.

Other causes of persistent local pain are due to damage to facial structures, such as the temporomandibular joint and orbital and nasal structures. Specialist advice may be needed.

Late headache

Some patients do not report significant headache to begin with and then complain of it later. The possible structural causes will need to be explored. If these have been excluded, some have maintained that a headache coming on later in this way cannot be due to the injury. However, usually it will be found that the patient has been able to cope with the restricted lifestyle of convalescence, but when they try to return to full activity they find they cannot cope. The headache which they then develop is usually of the fatigue type, and can be managed by reduction of demands and stress.

Persistent headache

The headache that some patients complain of does not fit comfortably into any of the varieties described above. Like the fatigue headaches it is usually felt throughout the head, though it may be localized to one area, perhaps the site of the original injury. It may be a constant ache or feel more like a tight band round the head. Throbbing is uncommon but may occur with exercise. It differs from the usual fatigue headache by being present often on waking, coming on at any time of the day, and not depending on activity, though usually it does get worse with fatigue or stress. It only responds fitfully to common analgesics; sometimes a patient may use these to excess and make the condition worse. On investigation there is no important contribution from the other sources of headache, though there may be some scalp or cervical soreness due to tension and muscle spasm.

In some patients the headache is directly connected with stress. They may have been responsible for the accident, others may have been injured, and there may be a question of legal liability. There is often financial loss, compensation to be negotiated, or a claim to be arranged.

Many patients become depressed if the headache continues without improvement. Especially when there is a history of depression in the past or of personal problems, this may progress to a significant clinical depression and even to suicidal ideation. If this situation seems to be developing a psychiatric opinion will be needed.

In an occasional patient the pain may be simulated, but this is likely to have been detected in a patient who has been properly investigated and particularly if they have been observed over a period of time.

Unfortunately the headache may sometimes continue in patients who are genuinely anxious to get back to a normal productive life.

Treatment should follow the general management of the PCS described in Chapter 9. It is important to start as soon as possible before the patient loses heart, and that there should be a positive and confident approach. An antidepressant should be used, working up to the maximum dose that allows the patient to carry on with normal activities without impairing cognitive function. A tricyclic antidepressant such as amitriptyline will suit most patients in whom the headache is the most prominent feature; others where stress and depression are major factors may do better with fluoxetine. A regular structured programme of activity should be arranged and supervised, even if it starts with a very short time each day. The patient's physical condition has often deteriorated and it is desirable that there should be a graduated exercise programme. Other support measures such as counselling, meditation techniques, and acupuncture should be enlisted but should not divert attention from the main programme.

Comment

A great deal has been written about post-traumatic headache. Cartlidge, reporting on a major prospective study of head injury in the 1970s, expressed a view that is still current that headache is the most frequent of all sequelae of head injury, causes protracted distress and incapacity, and taxes the resourcefulness and sometimes the patience of the carers. He said that together with dizziness, irritability, and poor concentration it formed the 'post-concussion syndrome', but that headache was undoubtedly the most consistent and troublesome feature. This properly emphasizes the importance of headache to both the patient and the doctor but it probably puts too much weight on headache as the primary cause of disability. As described above, many headaches are secondary to other conditions, whose management will do much to deal with the headache. We have found that often it is not so much the headache that is the cause of distress and incapacity as the inability to cope with the everyday tasks of living. When the patient has grasped this the headache often becomes less important to them.

As mentioned earlier in this section, the absence of physical signs – and perhaps the frustration of the doctor – can suggest that the symptoms are neurotic in origin or may even be simulated. It is certainly true that patients often emphasize their headache. The consequences of head injury are difficult for the lay person to understand and they will use the one piece of currency that they have to communicate their problems to the doctor.

Further reading

Barcellos, S. and Rizzo, M. (1996). Post-traumatic headaches. In *Head injury and postconcussive syndrome*, (ed. M. Rizzo and D. Tranel), pp. 139–75. Churchill Livingstone, New York.

A very full discussion of the types of headache and mechanisms, and of pharmacological management, with full references. Academic rather than practical.

Barnat, M. R. (1986). Post traumatic headache patients. *Headache*, **26**, 271–7; 332–8.
A study of the demographics and psychology of patients with post-traumatic headache.

Cartlidge, N. E. F. and Shaw, D. A. (1981). *Head injury*. W.B. Saunders, London.
This contains a careful analysis of symptoms in patients followed for several years – illuminating, though the conclusions may be questioned in the light of the understanding of symptoms that has come from developments in neuropsychology.

Haas, D. C. and Lourie, H. (1988). Trauma-triggered migraine: an explanation for common neurological attacks after mild had injury. *Journal of Neurosurgery*, **68**, 181–8.

Hopkins, A. (ed.) (1988). *Headache. Problems in diagnosis and management.* W.B. Saunders, London.
This has a chapter on headache after cranial trauma by Reginald Kelly and other sections on possible causes, with a consideration of the contribution of the psychiatrist. Though published in 1988, the information has not dated.

Kelly, R. E. (1986). Post-traumatic headache. In *Handbook of clinical neurology, Volume 48, Headache.* Elsevier, Amsterdam.
Another entry to Kelly's analysis of post-traumatic headache, which may be more easily obtained than Hopkins (1988).

Matthews, W. B. (1972). Footballer's migraine. *British Medical Journal*, **i**, 326–7.
This classic short article drew attention to trauma-triggered migraine.

VISUAL SYMPTOMS

Introduction

Major head injuries may damage the optic nerves, chiasm, tract, or cortex and cause clear-cut defects of vision; lesions of the third, fourth, and sixth nerves will result in a characteristics diplopia. Visual symptoms also occur after mild injury. They are usually less well defined, such as blurring of vision, mild diplopia in central gaze, and photophobia. In one series of consecutive patients with mild head injury admitted to hospital overnight, symptoms were present in 6 per cent at six weeks and 3 per cent at a year. They were one of the complaints in about 20 per cent of people referred to the authors' clinic with post-concussion problems, and remained a significant symptom at one year in about 5 per cent. Because the findings on examination may be indefinite there has been a tendency to regard the symptoms as functional.

Here we will describe a routine of clinical examination of a patient with visual symptoms following a mild head injury, and will discuss diagnosis and possible mechanisms. Management can be straightforward or reference to an ophthalmologist may be needed.

Routine clinical examination

When the patient is first seen they may be wearing dark glasses or turn away from the light because of photophobia. External signs of damage to the eye or orbit should be looked for, palpating the inferior orbital margin and testing the sensation in the distribution of the infraorbital nerve.

Measure the visual acuity in either eye at 6 m with Snellen or similar charts, making sure that they are well lit, and test close vision with reading charts. Do this first without correction and then repeat with glasses if the patient uses them. If acuity is reduced, repeat the tests with trial lenses if they are available, or with the patient viewing the charts through a pinhole.

The fundi and optic discs should be examined. Abnormalities in patients with mild head injury are rare, but occasionally a blow to the orbital region results in retinal damage. Direct and consensual pupil reactions should be tested.

Test the visual field of each eye. With the patient seated 1 m from the examiner, test peripheral vision with finger movements at 60° from fixation. Examine central vision with small (about 3 mm) white and red balls – a dressmaker's pin, perhaps – on a black wand, which are moved in a plane half way between patient and examiner. With the patient fixing on the examiner's eye, first check that the examiner's and patient's blind spots coincide, giving a marker for about 17° from fixation, then check that the object can be seen throughout the central field, up to around 20° from fixation for the red, when the colour should be lost, and 30° when the white should be lost. If there appears to be a defect, such as a scotoma due to retinal damage or a peripheral or hemianopic loss, further charting on a Goldman or other perimeter will be needed.

Explore conjugate eye movements. When pursuit is normal the eyes should be able to follow a finger across the central 90° of the visual field in about three seconds with a smooth movement uninterrupted by saccades. Then test rapid movement from one target to another. Irregular pursuit or abnormal saccades are, however, unusual after mild injury. If there is a complaint of diplopia, note the direction of gaze which produces it.

Test accommodation and convergence by having the patient fix on an object which is moved in the midline towards the nose. A pencil held vertically may be used, or if possible an instrument such as the RAF rule. The distance at which the target blurs is the near point of accommodation. The point at which it becomes double, or the patient can converge no further and the eyes diverge, is the near point of convergence. Patients should be ale to maintain fusion up to about 7 cm from the bridge of the nose. With forced convergence of this sort there should be constriction of the pupils.

When there is diplopia after a mild head injury, unless it is due to damage to one of the oculomotor nerves, it is usually minor and it may be difficult to see any limitation of eye movement; it will then be necessary to depend on the patient's report on the displacement of the images. They should be asked to look in the direction in which the images are most separated. The image which is furthest displaced in this direction is derived from the affected eye, and this can be identified by covering one eye and noting which image disappears. Patients often find it difficult to be sure about this, especially when there is central diplopia. The simplest solution is to use goggles with a red filter over the right eye and a green filter over the left. The patient views a torch bulb and is asked to describe the relations of the red and green images as their eyes follow the light as it moves round the field of vision. Normally the red and green images fuse in all directions; when there is diplopia they separate in a characteristic way.

Common abnormalities

Blurring of vision

Intermittent blurring of vision is common in the first few days after mild head injury. Vision cannot be improved with lenses or a pinhole. Patients are usually able to distinguish this from double vision, and the examiner will find that occluding one eye does not help. In most cases the blurring clears in a week or so. The nature and cause of the blurring is uncertain.

Blurring may persist. This is most often seen in people who are in their 40s or older. On examination it is commonly found that reading acuity is reduced but distant vision is normal, and that reading acuity can be restored with suitable lenses. Usually there is no improvement in acuity with time, and it appears that the injury has resulted in an early presbyopia, presumably from the weakening of compensatory mechanisms.

Younger people may also complain of blurring of vision. In some cases distance vision is impaired with close vision being normal, the patient in fact becoming myopic. The cause appears to be spasm of accommodation and if this is the case, cycloplegic refraction, with the ciliary muscle paralysed, will be normal. This is usually a temporary condition and vision can be expected to return to normal after a few weeks or months.

In a few cases blurring persists without the cause being evident. Further examination using tests of contrast sensitivity or visual evoked potentials have been done in these patients, but so far no definite cause has been found in most cases. Improvement may follow careful refraction and corrective lenses. There may be abnormalities in neuropsychological tests, and it is possible that impairment of central processing may play a part. Often no explanation can be found, sometimes with the result that the symptom is labelled as functional.

Diplopia

There may be definite diplopia due to damage to the third or sixth nerves, though this is rare after a mild injury. Damage to the fourth nerve, often partial, does occasionally occur after mild injury. When complete there is diplopia on looking downwards and away from the side of the lesion, with limited adduction of the ipsilateral eye. With red and green glasses the image from the affected eye will then be below and to the outer side of the other. The patient may compensate for the diplopia by tilting their head away from the lesion. The lesion may be partial, when the diplopia may be difficult to characterize, and in this case the compensatory inclination of the head may be a useful clue.

Probably the commonest form is a mild double vision present in central gaze, often only coming on when the patient is tired. On examination there is slight horizontal separation of the images; red and green glasses will show that each image derives from the contralateral eye. This is due to a weakness of convergence, presumably of central origin.

Orbital fractures may result in diplopia, commonly on looking upwards and due to tethering of the inferior rectus in a fracture of the floor of the orbit; it is likely to be accompanied by loss of sensation in the area of the infraorbital nerve.

A strabismus which was present in childhood may recur in an adult after mild injury, presumably due to impairment of compensation. It usually clears spontaneously after a month or two.

Photophobia

Photophobia is common, even with indoor lighting and especially with fluorescent lights. The mechanism is uncertain and the severity sometimes does not match that of other symptoms, particularly the cognitive ones, and some patients continue to need dark glasses when they have otherwise recovered.

Visual field abnormalities

Sharp cut defects will be found after mild injury only if there has been an orbital fracture involving the region of the optic canal, or a direct injury to the globe with perhaps a retinal tear, such as can occur in boxing injuries. Though few patients may show such a field defect in the routine testing we have described, in a considerable number there will be subtle impairment of visual function in the peripheral fields. If reaction times to visual stimuli are measured they may be increased relative to those in the central fields. Both sides may be abnormal; when only one is affected it may correspond to a presumed area of damage as indicated by defects of verbal or spatial function.

The impairment of function in peripheral fields helps to explain the poor avoidance described in the section on dizziness, and is of practical importance in deciding whether a patient is ready to resume activities such as driving.

Stereopsis, depth perception

The ability to judge distances and to relate objects to each other is provided by a complex mechanism involving both the convergence mechanism of the eye and higher visual centres. The higher centres operate on the relations between objects, their shapes, and their sizes and depend on central processing ability. As it is known that both parts of this mechanism may be affected by mild injury it is not surprising that depth perception can be affected. Clinically this is not often identified as a problem, but it plays a part in difficulties in orientation and avoidance. If it is suspected that there may be a significant impairment, the ophthalmologist can arrange for investigation.

Cortical blindness

This may occur in children after a mild injury and is described in Chapter 11. The onset may be immediate or delayed for minutes or up to an hour or so. Pupil reflexes are usually normal, and sight returns after minutes to hours.

Comment

There is no doubt that visual disturbances are frequent after mild head injury. Blurring of vision is common in the early days and there may be diplopia; photophobia may continue when other symptoms have cleared.

Except when there has been damage to the eye or the orbit these symptoms must be of central origin. They can occur in three ways:

1. Where mechanisms compensating for previous abnormalities have been impaired. This is seen when the injury results in an early presbyopia and when adjustment for childhood strabismus breaks down.

2. Where the mechanisms of accommodation and convergence are impaired. The brainstem centres which coordinate the focus and direction of each eye on fixed and moving targets, and adjust the size of the pupil, are very complex and it is easy to understand how they could be upset by the small brainstem lesions that we know can occur in mild injury. The disturbance of accommodation which results in the appearance of myopia, and of convergence, which cause central diplopia, must be due

to disturbance of this system. In some cases the mechanism reorganizes itself in time, but it may remain impaired.

3. Where higher cerebral function is affected. As well as depending on a sharply focused image congruent on the two retinae, visual perception also depends on a chain of higher functions at various levels. In severe injury damage to them can have a variety of consequences, from field defects to visual agnosia. In mild injury, more subtle defects may be the cause of persistent blurring or impaired depth perception.

The origin of photophobia is uncertain. It may lie in the brainstem, perhaps being associated with the regulation of pupillary size. Though it may be central, as is probably the case in noise intolerance, it does not necessarily improve when other central functions do.

It is often held that the less easily explained visual symptoms are a part of the behavioural disorder which may occur after mild head injury. Certainly similar problems with accommodation can occur when there has been no injury and against a background of personality disorder. It seems more likely, however, that in most cases the impairment of function is due to direct damage to brainstem structures. There are many reports in the literature of obvious and sometimes quite severe malfunction of the oculomotor nuclei after head injuries which appeared to be trivial, often when there had been no loss of consciousness. It is easy to conceive how the complex mechanisms of pursuit, convergence, and accommodation could be disturbed in subtle ways by similar but less severe injuries.

Visual symptoms can, however, be functional. A false complaint of major loss of vision in one eye can usually be detected by distracting the patient and forcing them to use the affected eye. A complaint of generally restricted visual fields – tunnel vision – is commoner. Examining the fields at 1 m and 3 m is likely to show the distant field smaller than the nearer one, plainly not physiological.

Management

Most of the visual symptoms seen in the early stages are mild and will clear after a week or two without specific treatment. When they persist, specialist advice will be needed. Refraction with and without cycloplegics will show whether blurring of vision is due to problems with accommodation. Diplopia can be more exactly categorized, spectacles with prisms or orthoptic treatment may be helpful, and occasionally ocular muscle surgery may be needed. When there is continued unexplained blurring, further investigation with measurement of contrast sensitivity and visually evoked potentials may make the situation more clear, though perhaps not add to treatment possibilities. In cases where no specific cause for symptoms can be found, management will consist of the general system of support and the expectation that the problem will slowly regress with the passage of time.

Further reading

Standard ophthalmic texts may be consulted. Articles worth reading that are specifically concerned with changes in minor injury are listed below.

Jefferson, A. (1961). Ocular complications of head injury. *Transactions of the Ophthalmological Society of the United Kingdom*, **81**, 595–612.
 Of interest as it includes descriptions of complex disturbances of the brainstem mechanisms resulting from minor head injury.
Kowal, L. (1992). Ophthalmic manifestations of head injury. *Australian and New Zealand Journal of Ophthalmology*, **20**, 35–40.
 This gives a practical account of most of the problems met with.
Mishra, A. V. and Digre, K. B. (1996). Neuro-ophthalmologic disturbances in head injuries. In *Head injuries and postconcussion syndrome*, (ed. M. Rizzo and D. Tranel). Churchill Livingstone, New York.
 This text is referred to in other chapters, and if available is worth consulting on visual problems.

ANOSMIA AND AGEUSIA

Introduction

The sense of smell is permanently affected in around 20 per cent of people with a severe head injury and a post-traumatic amnesia of more than 24 h. Loss is less common after milder injuries, but in one series was present at the first examination in some 8 per cent with PTA of less than 1 h and in 3 per cent of people who did not lose consciousness. When sophisticated methods of testing are used, the incidence of partial impairment may be greater.

Mechanisms and clinical features

Damage is most likely when there have been facial injuries or an occipital or vertex impact. There are three common mechanisms. Anterior cranial fossa fractures and facial injuries can damage the olfactory plate and its nerves. The nasal bones and mucosa can be distorted and block the airflow over an undamaged olfactory epithelium. An occipital impact can result in a backward shift of the brain which snaps the olfactory tracts or shears off the olfactory bulbs. Probably much less commonly, cortical damage may interfere with the central processing of olfactory sensation.

Recovery occurs in about half of the patients with mild head injury who have anosmia when first seen. It is more likely when the loss has been due to nasal blockage, if this clears spontaneously or with treatment. Probably there is little chance of recovery when the olfactory tracts or bulbs have been damaged. In practical terms, in an unselected group if recovery is to take place it will occur within 3 months in 75 per cent of cases, and only very rarely after 2 years.

Taste sensation depends largely on smell, and this will be grossly affected when there is anosmia, leaving only the appreciation of sweet, sour, salt, and bitter, which is mediated by receptors in the tongue through the trigeminal and glossopharyngeal nerves. Loss of taste without the loss of smell is uncommon. However, like anosmia, it can occur after a relatively minor injury. In 18 cases of ageusia without anosmia, the PTA was less than 24 h in 10. The pathology is uncertain. Damage to the chorda tympani or to the glossopharyngeal nerve may be responsible; a central lesion has been suggested.

Smell and taste loss may be followed by dysgeusia, when there is either a spontaneous abnormal taste sensation or one provoked by the sight of food or taste on the tongue. The sensation is almost always unpleasant.

Investigation

At the first interview after a mild head injury, the patient should always be asked about their ability to taste and smell. They should be asked whether they can tell when coffee is brewing or bacon cooking, or whatever food preparation is appropriate for them, and then whether they have experienced faecal or unpleasant smells without knowing where they came from. The sense of smell should then be tested. Useful materials are coffee beans, oil of cloves, lemon and almond essences, and tar. They should be in opaque bottles and presented to each nostril separately. Lingual taste may be tested by soaking a small cotton wool swab with salt or sugar solution or diluted vinegar and applying it to either side of the tongue.

The patient's report of loss of smell may sometimes be suspected. A very strong smell may then be tried, or one which could be expected to elicit an involuntary response. Note, however, that tears do not indicate perception of a smell, and that strong smells such as ammonia may stimulate the nasal mucosa and provoke tears by a reflex through the trigeminal nerve. Anosmia associated with loss of taste on the tongue may suggest dissimulation, but as we noted above it is possible for both sensations to be lost.

Management

Loss of smell and taste is a serious disability. Enjoyment of food, a major pleasure for most people, is usually affected. Eating habits may change, and loss of weight or dietary deficiencies can occur. Dysgeusia is uncommon, but can be more disturbing than loss of taste, as it can inhibit the eating of necessary foods. These losses can be a major factor in the onset of depression.

If the patient uses gas for cooking or heating, they may not notice leaks and it may be advisable to change to electricity. Their house should be well supplied with smoke detectors. A number of occupations depend on smell for their operation (food handling in particular), and others for safety (painting, fibreglass, and plastic fabricating and other trades where solvents are used). People in these trades will often need to change occupations.

Further reading

Coty, R. L., Shaman, P., Kimmelman, C. P., and Dann, M. S. (1984). University of Pennsylvania smell identification test: a rapid quantitative olfactory function test for the clinic. *Laryngoscope*, **94**, 176–8.
  Of interest if looking for more sophisticated tests.
Sumner, D. (1964). Post-traumatic anosmia. *Brain*, **87**, 107–20.
  Though more than 30 years old, this paper remains a classic.

DIZZINESS, IMPAIRED BALANCE, AND VERTIGO

Introduction

One or more of this group of symptoms is present in a high proportion of people recovering from head injury, both mild and more severe. In a consecutive group of patients who had had a mild head injury 15 per cent complained of dizziness six weeks after the accident and 5 per cent a year later (Rutherford *et al.* 1978). Twenty per cent of 250 MHI patients referred to the authors' clinic with PCS complained of one of these symptoms, as well as those relating to other systems. In the majority the symptoms clear spontaneously in a few weeks, but in some they persist and can be a major source of disability.

Clinical features

To begin with patients will commonly refer to most of these symptoms as 'dizziness'. The first step will be to have them describe the symptoms more fully, when they will usually fall into one of the following groups.

(1) Unreal sensations. Patients will say that they feel out of touch with their surroundings, sometimes as if they were walking around with-

out touching the ground. This is common in the first few days after injury and may persist for a week or two, even when the patient has been fit enough to return to work. Later on it may be described by patients with other PCS problems when they have become stressed and feel unable to cope with events.

(2) Minor instability. In situations where a sense of position is needed, such as going down stairs or standing at an edge with nothing to hold on to, patients may feel insecure.

(3) Poor balance. The patient is aware that their balance is unsteady when they are standing or walking, and they say that it is usually much worse in the dark.

(4) Vertigo. The patient feels they are moving, usually rotating but also falling backwards or occasionally veering sideways. Early after the injury this can be spontaneous and severe, with nausea and vomiting. Later it is generally brought on by any movement of the head. A common pattern is rotatory vertigo on getting out of bed. Attacks may continue for a minute or more, and usually cannot be provoked again until the patient has remained still for a while. Vertigo may also be provoked by looking upwards without moving the head, or with a variety of visual stimuli such as watching the passing countryside out of a train window. Nausea commonly accompanies the vertigo.

(5) Poor avoidance. The patient bumps into the side of doorways or into other people in the street. Balance is otherwise unaffected.

Basis of symptoms

Impaired information processing

This affects the patient's general appreciation of surroundings and events and their response to them. This is likely to be the major cause of the feelings of floating and disorientation seen in the early days after injury, and is probably responsible for the minor instability and insecurity when there is no obvious vestibular dysfunction. There is often a slow reaction time to visual stimuli in the peripheral fields, and this is likely to be at least part of the cause of the poor avoidance situation (see later in this chapter and Chapter 8).

Damage to the vestibular system

This is the most important cause of this group of symptoms. The vestibular system relies on the three semicircular canals, arranged mutually at right angles, and on the utricle and saccule. These communicate with each other and are filled with endolymph. In each canal there is a dilatation into which a group of hair cells protrudes. Acceleration of the head in the plane of the canal creates a current in the endolymph, deflects the hairs, and sends a signal via the vestibular nerve. In the utricle and saccule there are tufts of hair cells covered by a gelatinous matrix in which are embedded crystals of calcium carbonate, the otoconia. The pressure of the crystals on the hair cells alters with the position of the head and signals its orientation. It is important to note that in both systems the response to stimuli fatigues rapidly.

It is easy to see, when there are severe injuries such as fractures of the base of the skull, how these delicate structures can be disrupted and how vestibular responses can become deranged. This will show at first in severe and continuous vertigo and nausea, lasting for some days until the vestibular system adjusts; it usually then becomes intermittent and occurs only when there is head movement. In mild head injury there may be similar but less severe symptoms to begin with. In some patients symptoms continue, with vertigo on certain positions or movements of the head. The picture is similar to that of benign positional vertigo, which may occur when there has been no obvious trauma. In either case the symptoms are usually due to debris rolling around the semicircular canals, either otoconia that have dislodged from the gelatinous matrix or, possibly, minor bleeding or other damage when there has been trauma. Occasionally it can be shown that the membrane sealing the membranous labyrinth at the circular or oval windows has been torn. Perilymph then leaks and unbalances the canals and saccule and utricle, which produces vertigo.

Cervical causes

There are many afferents from the cervical structures which reach the vestibular nuclei, and musculoskeletal lesions in the neck can result in vertigo.

Central causes

Though it is uncommon, even mild head injury can damage central cerebellar connections and produce incoordination of the hand or leg (see later in this chapter), and so disturb balance. There is also some evidence that instability of the trigeminovascular system may be involved (see Chapter 3).

Secondary distress

As we have said elsewhere, continued disability due to head injury and the anxiety and stress it produces may result in the growth of minor symptoms into major problems, and slight dizziness and balance impairment may become serious complaints in this way, perhaps inducing other syndromes such as chronic hyperventilation.

Examination

In the neurological examination special attention should be paid to signs of cerebellar dysfunction, for nystagmus in lateral and upward gaze, in impairment of finger–nose testing and rapid repetitive movement, and for incoordination in heel–shin testing in the legs. The external auditory meatus should be checked for signs of injury and tests of hearing will show if there is any gross loss which might be associated with a vestibular lesion.

Balance may be assessed by a sequence of tests:

(1) standing balanced with feet apart, together, and one in front of the other, with eyes open and eyes shut;

(2) standing on one leg, with eyes open and eyes shut;

(3) hopping on either foot;

(4) walking in a straight line, with eyes open and then with eyes shut;

(5) walking heel–toe;

(6) running 10 m.

In specialist otology units a scoring system may be used to record the results of these tests, but for the present purposes a narrative description is adequate.

When there is typical vertigo it may have been provoked by the tests performed so far. If not, an attempt should be made to provoke it. The ordinary range of head movements, especially looking upwards, may do this, or persistent or repeated lateral gaze. The formal test which is most useful to someone who is not an otologist is the Dix–Hallpike manoeuvre. The patient is placed on an examining couch so that when they lie down their shoulders are over the end of the bed. They first sit up, and then with the examiner steadying their head they lie down swiftly with their head coming to rest inclined some 45° downwards and turned to one side. A positive response is reproduction of the vertigo, and usually the onset after 3 s or so of nystagmus. The response is more marked when the head is turned with the vestibular system at fault downwards.

When the vertigo is severe and persistent, further investigation by an otologist is advisable, and caloric responses, electronystagmography, and balance platform testing may be indicated. The interpretation and possible actions in response to these tests is beyond the scope of this book, and it will be necessary to rely on the otologist's special knowledge.

Diagnosis

Unreal sensations

When these occur in the first week or two after injury and there is no
more than mild instability and no true vertigo, the cause can be taken
to be general impairment of processing and the symptoms will disappear
as this improves. Occurring later, in the presence of continuing symptoms, particularly when there is distress from vertigo, chronic habitual
hyperventilation will need to be considered.

Minor instability

The sense of instability in circumstances in which normal people may
feel that they would have to pay attention to their balance and the relative mildness of the symptoms are typical. The examination may show
some mild impairment of balance, but this is only slightly more marked
when the eyes are closed. Some impairment of concentration and attention is likely. In the absence of other abnormalities the diagnosis can rest
on these findings.

Loss of balance

The history will be of loss of balance and an unsteady gait, which is
worse in the dark. On examination, performance on the tests of balance
will be impaired, and will be worse with the eyes closed. There is, however, no history of vertigo and none on provocation. In the milder cases it
can be taken that there has been some damage to the vestibular system
which is likely to clear spontaneously. When the symptoms are marked,
especially in older people, and if on examination there are signs of cerebellar dysfunction, it may be necessary to consider other pathology, and a
CT scan and full neurological investigation may be advisable.

Vertigo

The patient's description of the symptoms will usually leave little doubt of
the diagnosis of damage to the vestibular system, and the tests of balance
and the provocative manoeuvres should confirm it. Again, in older
people, cerebrovascular disease may need to be considered, or Ménière's
syndrome, and if there are doubts referral to an otologist is wise.

Management

When the dizziness is mild, explanation of its origin and the general support and management appropriate to the head injury will generally be

sufficient. The condition will usually cease to be disturbing, and gradually regress.

When there are significant problems with balance and coordination, without evidence of other pathology, a programme of exercises with a physiotherapist will be helpful.

Mild vertigo is common in the early days after head injury and usually settles spontaneously. If there is significant nausea, prochlorperazine (Stemetil) or similar medication for a time will help most patients. Often for some time, when the more severe vertigo has stopped, mild attacks will continue on one or two occasions in the day, particularly on getting out of bed, and this is usually best treated by support and reassurance; long term medication should be avoided.

When the vertigo persists and is mild it may be a useful and conservative treatment to provoke it deliberately a number of times a day. This may allow the vestibular system to become habituated to stimuli and respond less. It may be sufficient to tell the patient to repeat the movements that bring on the vertigo as often as they can, at times when this does not interfere with their daily activity. If this is not effective a formal set of exercises may be useful. Those originally devised by Cawthorne are commonly used:

Begin in a sitting position, then
   lie flat on your back
   roll to the left side
   roll to the right side
   lie flat on your back
   sit up.
Now stand:
   turn to the right
   turn to the left.
Sit again:
   put your nose on your left knee
   place your right ear on your right shoulder
   put your nose on your right knee
   place your left ear on your left shoulder.
While sitting:
   turn your head sharply to the left
   turn your head sharply to the right
   repeat these two bending forward
   repeat while going from sitting to standing
   repeat as you move your head forward
   repeat as you move your head backward.
Still sitting:
   hang your head between your legs, turning to the left
   sit up
   hang your head turning to the right
   sit up

hang your head in the middle between your legs
sit up.

The patient should select the six exercises which provoke the most severe symptoms and perform these for 10 minutes twice a day.

If the symptoms are more severe or fail to improve with these measures, referral to an otologist is advisable. We have said earlier that it is probable that most persistent vertigo is caused by the movement of displaced otoconia or other debris in the semicircular canals. Techniques have been developed in otology in which by a series of head movements – the canalith repositioning manoeuvres, CNP – this material is manoeuvred into the vestibule of the system where it ceases to disturb vestibular function. In some of the cases in which the Cawthorne type of exercise has helped it is probable that this, rather than habituation, is responsible for the improvement. Occasionally the otologist may find a structural lesion in the ear, such as a perilymphatic fistula, which may be suitable for operative treatment.

Lastly, patients with troublesome vertigo lead a restricted life and usually take little exercise; a well designed fitness programme in a reputable gym may be helpful.

Further reading

Brandt, T. (1994). Therapy for benign positional vertigo, revisited. *Neurology,* **44**, 796–800.
  A review article.
Fitzgerald, D. C. (1996). Head trauma: hearing loss and dizziness. *Journal of Trauma: Injury, Infection and Critical Care,* **40**, 488–96.
  This review article goes into detail on the pathology and management of dizziness and vertigo and is a good source of further references.
Rutherford, W. H., Merrett, J. D., and McDonald, J. R. (1978). Symptoms at one year following concussion from minor head injuries. *Injury,* **10**, 225–30.
  We have referred to this and their preceding paper often, as a source of information on the incidence of clinical features after mild head injury.

HEARING

At follow-up visits after mild head injury some patients complain of deafness. Usually it is in one ear only and there has been evidence of some local trauma such as bruising around the ear or bleeding into the meatus. There may have been a fracture of the base of the skull, though this would be unusual in an otherwise mild injury.

Deafness may have been present before the accident and only noted afterwards, so that other possible causes should be looked for. These may have been running ears and otitis media as a child, industrial noise, or the use of firearms. It should be asked whether the deafness is continuous, and whether it is associated with tinnitus or vertigo.

The meatus and eardrum should be examined, wax and debris being cleaned out if necessary. Acuity in each ear is tested by the ability to detect a whisper. Bone and air conduction are assessed with low and high pitch tuning forks.

With this history and basic examination it can be determined whether there is likely to be significant deafness and a provisional diagnosis of middle or inner ear origin can be made. Pure tone and speech audiometry will help to confirm the diagnosis, and if there is significant deafness, referral to an otologist will be needed.

Quite often the patient will complain of deafness but on testing, auditory acuity in either ear is normal. They will usually confirm that they do not notice the deafness when talking with a single person and in quiet surroundings. When there is a general conversation with several people, and typically in gatherings such as a cocktail party, they can make out little of what people are saying. Identifying and holding on to one line of thought under these circumstances requires substantial concentration; patients who complain of these symptoms will be found to have a depressed capacity for processing information (see Chapter 8). They should be reassured that as this improves their 'deafness' will recover.

Further reading

The review article by Fitzgerald (1996) referred to in the section on dizziness is a useful source of further information.

OTHER FINDINGS

Impaired coordination

Incoordination that was obvious, either of hand or leg, would not be compatible with a diagnosis of mild head injury. However, some patients will report that one hand is clumsy, and often that they tend to drop things. If they have special manual skills they may feel that the hand is just not performing properly, though ordinary tasks are managed with little difficulty. More rarely one leg may feel clumsy and liable to trip.

On clinical examination, power and reflexes will probably be symmetrical, but in tests of coordination such as the finger–nose test there may be some tremor or uncertainty on the affected side and difficulty with repetitive movements; these may sometimes have a 'flapping' quality. Again, heel–shin coordination may be slightly impaired and repeated toe-tapping irregular. It is unlikely that there will be nystagmus or other sign of a cerebellar lesion.

The incoordination can be assessed in more detail by having the patient perform one of a group of formal tests of coordination, usually timed, such as placing pegs into holes in a pegboard. More elaborate procedures in which movements are recorded electronically may be available.

Imaging is unlikely to show any abnormality. However, in autopsies there have been microscopic lesions seen in the superior cerebellar peduncle on one side, apparently where it has impinged on the edge of the tentorium at the moment of impact, and such lesions could well be the cause of this syndrome. Another element in the pattern of incoordination may be the slowing of response time, which can occur in mild injury. This is probably the factor responsible for the poor performance in tests in which there is an element of choice as well as of coordination, such as the digit symbol test mentioned in Chapter 8.

In most cases of impaired coordination occurring after mild head injury the disability is not great, though highly skilled people may be disadvantaged. In them and where the incoordination is more marked, a well planned programme of exercise is likely to be helpful, though progress may be slow.

Cervical spine injuries

Neck injuries commonly accompany mild head injuries, and their part in causing headache has been discussed. There may also be shoulder and arm weakness and disturbance of sensation. Their management is outside our scope here, and specialist help should be sought.

POST-TRAUMATIC EPILEPSY

Introduction

Post-traumatic epilepsy is an important complication of major head injury. It can also occur as a result of a mild head injury, though the incidence is probably little different from that in the population as a whole. Nevertheless some people who have had a mild head injury do present with seizures, often with features which make diagnosis difficult.

Clinical features

Immediate seizures

Occasionally, immediately after an injury which would otherwise be classed as mild, before the recovery of consciousness, there may be one or a series of convulsions. These may be generalized, or one side or one limb can be mainly involved. When consciousness returns there may be some slight weakness if there have been focal features, but recovery is likely to be swift and uncomplicated. Some patients have cognitive problems later, though probably not more often than would be expected after an injury of comparable severity if there had been no seizure. The important point is that if when the patient is examined a day or two after the injury there is no persistent abnormality, further seizures are most unlikely, and full investigation and prophylactic medication is not indicated (McRory *et al.* 1997).

Early seizures

Around 2 per cent of patients seen at hospital and classified as having a mild head injury will have a seizure in the first seven days, more often in the first 24 h. In around half of them, CT will show an intracranial haemorrhage or a frontal or temporal parenchymal lesion and in these, not coming within our definition of a mild injury, the incidence of late seizures is of the order of 20 per cent. In those without a structural lesion the incidence is around 5 per cent. In children the incidence of seizure is higher, and there is a tendency to status epilepticus, which can be fatal; in Chapter 4 we commented on the need for decisive treatment.

Late seizures

The incidence of later seizures which occur in patients who have had an uncomplicated mild head injury is around 0.5 to 1 per cent, of the order of that in the general population. In 250 patients referred to the authors with persisting symptoms after mild head injury, there was a question of seizures in 6 per cent. They are most often simple or complex partial seizures. They may have the full complement of features, with an aura, stereotyped abnormal behaviour, impairment of consciousness, and post-ictal confusion, but often the episodes consist only of a period of absence followed by mild confusion, so that the patient's family may not appreciate that there is something wrong until several of these seizures have occurred.

Pseudoseizures may be seen after mild head injury. The more florid varieties may be recognized by the maintenance of consciousness, aimless and non-repetitive movements, and the variation of features from attack to attack. When the main features are an apparent absence and amnesia, the distinction on clinical grounds from a partial seizure may be impossible. When pseudoseizures are suspected, particular attention should be paid to the patient's past history and to sources of stress before and after the accident. A psychiatric opinion will be helpful. It should be remembered, however, that disturbed people can have genuine seizures.

Investigation

The first essential is a detailed account from the patient and those around them of when the seizures first occurred, what happens in them, and the frequency and any factors which seem to provoke them. The next step will be to consult with the clinical neurophysiologist on arranging EEG studies, which will include sleep recordings. Unfortunately, routine recordings often show no abnormality, in some series in 20–40 per cent of cases. When the clinical features are definite and the attacks frequent or severe enough to be a significant disability, further EEG studies will be needed. These may be long term ambulant EEG recording with telemetry or combined EEG and video recording. They will be necessary especially when the seizures are atypical or pseudoseizures are suspected. An MR scan may be helpful if it shows lesions in the temporal or subfrontal areas, those most likely to result in complex partial seizures. In some cases, where the clinical features seem typical and there are no abnormalities on investigation, a trial of anticonvulsants may be the most effective diagnostic tool.

Management

When there have been immediate seizures, and if, when the patient is seen a day or two after the injury, there is no neurological or cognitive abnormality, further seizures are most unlikely and full investigation or prophylactic medication are not indicated.

A seizure occurring in the first seven days must be investigated with a CT scan, to rule out a structural lesion. If one is found and treated, a period of prophylactic anticonvulsant medication is advisable. If no lesion is seen, the decision on medication will depend on the severity of the seizures and whether there were focal features at the time or later, and on the patient's social and employment situation and personal choice.

In the case of late seizures, when the pattern is typical and there is a definite EEG abnormality, anticonvulsants should be started. If the EEG is normal, but the clinical features are definite and there is a significant disability, a trial of anticonvulsants is reasonable. If the seizures stop, they were probably epileptic in origin, and medication should continue. If they do not stop, further investigation may be needed and consideration of the possible behavioural causes of pseudoseizures is needed.

The anticonvulsants most often used to begin with are carbamazepine and valproate. Patients with mild head injury often find that phenytoin increases their cognitive problems, so that it is not a drug of choice. Carbamazepine also may have this effect, but seems to be well tolerated in most people. If the seizures are not controlled by carbamazepine or valproate, one of the more recently introduced anticonvulsants may be indicated – gabapentin, lamotrigine, or vigabatrin. In such a case consultation with a neurologist familiar with these medications would be advisable.

If there have been definite seizures, or a suspicion that they might be occurring, the part played by other medication may be questioned. Tricyclics can provoke seizures with large doses, but these will rarely be used in the management of mild head injury. Fluoxetine and methylphenidate have no adverse effect. It would therefore be usual to continue other medication alongside the anticonvulsants.

Where the seizures have been definite and medication appears to have controlled them, eventually the question will arise whether treatment could be stopped. Usually this should not be considered until two years have passed. Certainly control must have been complete and probably there should be no EEG abnormalities. If it is then decided to stop, the medication should be reduced slowly over three or four weeks.

As well as the medical considerations, it is important to take into account the patient's social and employment situation. The initial restrictions on driving will probably have ceased after a period of control, and these will have to be reimposed until the epilepsy is again 'controlled'. In some occupations there are similar limitations. For financial and social reasons it may therefore be preferable not to stop medication until the conditions it imposes can be dealt with.

Further reading

Jennett, B. (1975). *Epilepsy after non-missile head injuries*, (2nd edn). Heinemann, London.
  This is a treasure house of information, still relevant.
Lee, S.-T. and Lui, T.-N. (1992). Early seizures after mild closed head injury. *Journal of Neurosurgery*, **76**, 435–9.
  A large number of patients and well controlled observations make this a useful study; it does not extend for more than six months after injury.
McRory, P. R., Bladin, P. F., and Berkovic, S. F. (1997). Retrospective study of concussive convulsions in elite Australian rules and rugby league footballers: phenomenology, aetiology and outcome. *British Medical Journal*, **314**, 171–4.

Though the subjects are limited, this thorough study should be applicable to other patients.

Yablon, S. A. (1993). Posttraumatic seizures. *Archives of Physical Medicine and Rehabilitation,* **74**, 983–1001.

This is a very thorough account of more recent thinking.

7
Imaging and other investigations

Introduction

The major imaging techniques do not play an important part in the long term management of mild head injury. In the acute stage a CT scan is likely to be done if recovery is not rapid or straightforward, and in the next six weeks or so if persistent headache or other symptoms make it necessary to rule out a subdural haematoma. When symptoms persist diagnosis is made essentially on the clinical history and the neuropsychological assessment. If there are, in addition, focal neurological features such as diplopia or atypical headache, CT or MR may be needed to exclude other pathology. However CT, MR, PET, and SPECT have been used extensively in research on the causes of the late effects of mild head injury, as described in the section on mechanisms and pathology.

In a different category, EEG is essential when there is a question of post-traumatic epilepsy. Other electrodiagnostic tests have been used in research, though with little practical outcome.

CT scans

The use of CT in the acute stage is described in the section on ED management. At a later stage, clinical signs may suggest the possibility of a gross lesion such as a chronic subdural haematoma or post-traumatic hydrocephalus, or of intercurrent pathology not related to the head injury, and a CT scan will then be appropriate. Apart from major lesions, small areas of cortical loss may be seen, particularly in the subfrontal and temporal areas.

MR scans

At the time of writing it is uncommon to use MR in the acute stage of MHI management. CT is quicker and cheaper, better tolerated by patients, and shows the sort of lesion which may need continued observation or surgery. MR is more likely to be used later when there are long term and perhaps unexpected problems of cognition or behaviour, when there is concern that there is a cause other than head injury, or when it would be helpful to establish a structural cause for an atypical group of symptoms.

If MR scans are made in the acute stage on an unselected group of patients who are well enough to be allowed home from the ED, some 10 per cent are likely to show an abnormality, either a minimal subdural bleed or a parenchymal lesion. In more severe cases, those admitted to hospital for less than three days and still within the definition of MHI, the incidence rises to around 25 per cent. The lesions are usually seen in the grey matter or at the grey–white junction, are located in the orbitofrontal and temporal areas, and are only occasionally parietal or occipital. Deeper lesions are uncommon, with their proportion increasing with the depth and length of coma.

When scans are repeated after a month or so the majority of the acute lesions will be much smaller or will have disappeared completely; around 10 per cent are likely to be still present at three months.

Functional MR, fMR, can indicate areas of alteration of blood flow and has been used to outline parts of the brain where there is neural activity in response to willed functions such as movement or speech. It offers the possibility of locating areas responsible for impaired function after MHI and may have a use in confirming the findings of SPECT. Its cost and complexity make it unlikely that it will be used as a routine tool.

When patients with long-standing post-concussion symptoms are examined, the incidence of MR lesions is very much higher, almost all showing multiple small areas of cortical loss.

The relation between the lesions seen on MR and the presence and nature of symptoms is variable. As mentioned in the section on pathology, deep lesions rather than cortical ones relate to the depth and duration of coma. Patients with more severe and lasting symptoms are likely to have more cortical lesions, but though they are mostly in the frontal and temporal regions, their position is not consistently where one would expect from the detailed neuropsychological findings. Again, the lesions tend not to correspond with the areas of abnormal perfusion seen in PET and SPECT scans.

PET and SPECT scans

PET scanning uses a compound which is involved in cerebral metabolism, such as glucose, labelled with a radionuclide which emits positrons; as the positrons are annihilated by collisions with electrons, gamma rays are emitted. Their location is registered by a battery of detectors around the head and presented as a diagram in the basal or coronal plane, as in a CT scan, with a colour code to show the intensity in each area. The possibility of exploring both metabolism and blood flow make this an attractive method, but the cost of the equipment and of supplying the short-lived radionuclides needed has restricted its use.

In SPECT scanning a technetium compound emitting gamma rays is injected intravenously and the location and intensity of radiation is measured and presented in a similar way as in CT and PET scans. The normal scan distinguishes grey and white matter by their different perfusion rates, and will show areas where perfusion is anomalous, usually reduced. Its disadvantages are the coarse anatomical resolution and the lack of precision in the measurements of perfusion. It is, however, much cheaper and more often available than the alternative PET scan.

Most of the reports of SPECT in MHI have dealt with the findings in patients whose symptoms have persisted for three months to several years. In these the incidence of abnormalities has been high, from 50 to 100 per cent, with an average of two lesions per patient. When MR has been done at the same time, the abnormal areas have usually not coincided. The frontal and temporal regions have been most often involved, but again there has been poor correspondence between the location of the abnormal perfusion and the site that would have been expected from the neuropsychological findings.

At the time of writing there has been only one systematic study of SPECT which has followed patients through from the acute stage to a year after injury. This study, by Jacobs *et al.* (1996), covered 136 patients. Half showed no SPECT abnormality and had no long term symptoms. The other half showed both clinical and SPECT abnormalities which diminished with time. At one year, 93 per cent had returned to normal, but of the remainder with persisting symptoms, all but one showed SPECT abnormalities.

In spite of the lack of precision in the anatomy and quantitation of SPECT changes there appears to be strong evidence that abnormalities of perfusion are frequent in the early days after MHI, and that when symptoms persist, perfusion abnormalities are likely to be present. What the place of the technique is in clinical practice is at present uncertain. It does not have the advantage of MR of being able to rule out other pathologies when the clinical picture is not typical. It does, however, do more than standard MR in providing visible evidence of abnormal physiology when this would be helpful; fMR techniques may, however, be able to give comparable and confirmatory information. A difficulty may be that unless sufficient cases are scanned there may not be enough experience to give an opinion on borderline cases.

EEG

In most patients the EEG recorded hours or a few days after a mild head injury is normal; in a few there are mild diffuse abnormalities such as a slight increase in slow activity. Again, recordings after a month or two may show some slight generalized abnormalities but these are marginally, if at all, more common than in the general population and do not correlate with clinical findings. Except when there is a question of post-traumatic epilepsy, the EEG is not helpful (see Chapter 6).

Evoked potential studies

Changes in the EEG after auditory, somatosensory, and visual stimuli can be recorded by computer averaging of the responses to a large number of trials.

Auditory brainstem responses are obtained from repeated clicks to one ear. Seven successive responses can be distinguished, from structures ascending through the brainstem to the cortex. The interval most often affected is that between the response of the cochlea and that of the superior olive, and in some patients this may be prolonged immediately after mild injury, and though in a minority this change may persist, it does not correlate with symptoms of dizziness or loss of balance.

Somatosensory evoked potentials are usually generated by stimulating the median nerve at the wrist. The cortical responses would be of most relevance, but in mild head injury they give little information and in general they cannot be distinguished from those in normal people. One, the P300 response, which may relate to focused attention, has, however, been found to be reduced in the early stages after mild head injury.

Visual evoked potentials with stimuli of a reversing chequerboard pattern may be useful in sorting out problems of visual impairment after injury, but do not contribute usefully to the general investigation of mild injury.

Though they play an important role in major head injury, especially in the acute stage, evoked potentials are not in general useful in managing mild head injury.

Further reading

Doezema, D., King, J. N., Tandberg, D., Espinosa, M. C., and Orrison, W. W. (1991). Magnetic resonance imaging in minor head injury. *Annals of Emergency Medicine*, **20**, 1281–5.
An account of MR in consecutive unselected cases fit enough to be managed at home.

Ichise, M., Chung, D.-G., Wang, P., Wotzman, G., Gray, B. G., and Franks, W. (1994). Technetium-99m-HMPAO SPECT, CT and MRI in the evaluation of patients with chronic traumatic brain injury: a correlation with neuropsychological performance. *Journal of Nuclear Medicine*, **35**, 217–26.

Deals with findings in long-standing symptoms in mild and more severe cases.

Jacobs, A., Put, E., Ingels, M., Put, T., and Bossuyt, A. (1996). One year follow-up of technetium-99m-HMPAO SPECT in mild head injury. *Journal of Nuclear Medicine*, **37**, 1605–9.

A very well designed study of SPECT in mild head injury.

Levin, H. S., Williams, D. H., Eisenberg, H. M., High, W. M. Jr., and Guinto, F. C. Jr. (1992). Serial MRI and neurobehavioural findings after mild to moderate closed head injury. *Journal of Neurology, Neurosurgery and Psychiatry*, **55**, 255–62.

Describes MR and neuropsychological findings in the shorter term, with useful comments on their relationship.

Schoenhuber, R. and Gentilini, M. (1989). Neurophysiological assessment in mild head injury. In *Mild head injury*, (ed. H. S. Levin, H. M. Eisenberg, and A. L. Benton). Oxford University Press, New York.

A short account of several techniques and their application in mild head injury.

8

Assessment of cognition and behaviour

Introduction

Of all the deficits affecting the patient with a severe head injury the behavioural and cognitive changes are usually the most difficult for the clinician to manage, and are those that researchers rate as the most difficult for families to cope with (Lezac 1996). This applies as much if not more to cases of mild head injury, because problems with memory and concentration and mood swings may be the only persistent after-effects. Thus the patients may appear to others to be fully recovered, yet continue to complain that they are forgetful, and that they get tired and irritable very quickly. Further, it may be difficult to accept their claim that they do have problems. They are generally very aware that they cope badly when they are tired, and may prepare themselves for the doctor's appointment by having a rest or a sleep, so that he or she sees them at their unrepresentative best.

In the second part of this chapter we will deal in detail with the analysis and assessment of the problems of cognition and behaviour which follow mild head injury. First, however, it is important to outline what we know about the most common of these deficits and examine how they impinge on the patient's ability to function in everyday life.

Common deficits after mild head injury

Information processing rate

There is always a finite time lag between information arriving at our sense receptors and the execution of the appropriate reaction to this information. Apart from the time it takes for the messages to be transmitted through the nervous system, there is also the time needed to make the decision as to what is the appropriate action to take. Thus the term refers both to the speed with which we are able to respond to new information and to the amount of this information that we can hold in our minds at the same time. Clearly these are two sides of the same coin, since if we can process one item at a normal rate, we can deal with a reasonable number of the same items in a finite time. There is always some limit to the amount of information that can be dealt with at once, and this limit varies over the lifespan. Thus a toddler has only limited processing space; if he is given a paper sweet to unwrap he will sit down to do this because he is not able to attend to keeping himself standing at the same time as dealing with the sweet. The limit, or 'channel capacity', is finite and there is always a limit to how much we can do at once and how quickly we can do it. The capacity increases gradually with age and has generally reached its maximum by the early teens. At the other end of the lifespan the channel capacity reduces, so that the elderly take longer to make decisions, and cannot cope with as much information as they used to.

There can also be a short term reduction in capacity. Alcohol intoxication reduces channel capacity, as does even a short period of sleep deprivation. Reduction also occurs with head injury, and it has been well established that even after mild head injury information processing ability is almost invariably reduced (Levin *et al.* 1989), and that in some cases the reduction persists for many weeks.

Effect of reduced information processing rate on everyday function

In the early period after MHI people complain that they cannot cope with crowds, with noise, or with more than one visitor at a time. This is a direct effect of reduced information processing ability. Normally we are able to participate in a group discussion, and can keep track of who said what and which arguments have already been advanced. After a head injury, by the time that the patient has analysed what one speaker has said and prepared their own comment the conversation is likely to have moved on. When there is also background noise to filter out, as in a large gathering, this will use up further processing capacity and reduce the ability to function even more.

Some environments are particularly difficult. Supermarkets typify information overload, even for people who are well. The shopper is bombarded with a mass of visual input, with goods deliberately displayed to be 'eye-catching'. They are also smothered with auditory input from other shoppers, from the inevitable 'muzak', and from the intrusive announcements on the public address system. Given that at the same time they have to locate the items on their shopping list and keep track of what they still have to find, it is not surprising that the MHI patient is likely to give up in dismay, burst into tears or lose their temper; certainly they will develop a headache.

It is easy to understand therefore why someone who is still having difficulty in processing information at normal speeds will have problems in coping with work or school if this has to be carried out in situations where there is an information overload. They will have this problem even if they have shown that they can carry out the cognitive functions that are needed when they are on their own in a quiet room. In the same way it is understandable that they may be able to carry out a number of discrete activities separately but be unable to combine them together. For example, as three separate exercises, a patient may be able to look up a number in the phone book, be able to repeat a seven-digit number, and to dial seven digits on the telephone. What they may not be able to do as a single exercise is to look up the number, remember it, and dial it without error.

Attention and concentration

Reduced information processing ability is also considered to be the basis of the problems with attention and concentration that are invariably reported in MHI (Levin *et al.* 1989).

There are several aspects to attention. Focused attention is the ability to concentrate on one aspect of the environment and ignore irrelevant and distracting stimulation. It is the skill we use when we read a book or listen to music and 'switch off' from the distractions around us. It is related to the 'cocktail party' effect, where we can move from group to group in a crowded party and tune in only to the conversation of the group we are in at the time. It can be taken that filtering out irrelevant information and ignoring distraction requires some processing space and that after a head injury the patient is not able to access the amount required. They are likely to describe this as 'not being able to concentrate enough to enjoy reading any more' or as 'not being able to cope with groups of people'.

Another aspect of attention which is directly related to information processing capacity is termed 'divided attention'. This is the ability to carry out two activities at the same time. In adults, activities such as breathing and heartbeat are of course automatic, but so are complex behaviours such as understanding and using language. Many activities such as driving a car can also become 'over-learned' and mostly automatic. Thus we are generally able to hold a conversation with a passenger at the same time as we steer the car over a familiar route. However, if there is an unusual amount of other information to deal with at the same time, such as a traffic emergency, both listening and talking to the passenger will cease. In the same way if, before their accident, the student with a mild head injury had been able to listen to a lecture and take notes at the same time, now they may find this difficult or impossible.

Concentration span, or the ability to sustain attention, is another aspect. This is the length of time that we can maintain our attention on a task, and it is reduced when the information processing rate is reduced.

The student with an MHI who can normally cope with a one hour lecture can find that they start to 'drift off' after only 10 minutes or so. Another aspect of the ability to sustain attention is vigilance, the ability to maintain one's concentration when infrequent targets have to be watched for. If one is placed in a situation where it is important to watch for events that only occur infrequently, after a time, vigilance can begin to wane and some events may be missed. This fall-off in vigilance can occur more quickly after MHI. Some activities make special demands on vigilance. As an example, though driving a car over a familiar route becomes fairly automatic, it requires a degree of vigilance to detect and react to the unexpected, such as a child chasing a ball across the road.

Interaction with fatigue and stress

We have emphasized already the importance of fatigue in limiting how well someone will function after a head injury. It has been established that in normal people the ability to process information is reduced after a period of sleep deprivation and when they are overtired. Thus it is not surprising that in patients with a mild head injury the ability to attend and concentrate will vary during the day, depending on their level of fatigue. Clinicians need to bear in mind that they may be seeing patients at an unrepresentative point in this cycle. They need to be aware that some patients will come after a sleepless night, whilst others know that they perform badly when they are tired and have a sleep before their appointment.

Stress also interacts with cognitive function. The effect of stress on behaviour follows the classic bell-shaped curve (Lezac 1996). A certain level of stress is needed to maintain motivation, but beyond the optimum it leads to a deterioration of organized function. Thus most people have some stress in their lives, which may fulfil a useful function. People who have had a head injury experience additional stress, from finding that activities they could normally carry out are now impossible and from coping with the personal and financial problems that this creates. This 'secondary' stress will make things even more difficult for them, and a vicious cycle of deterioration may become established. It is to prevent this that help with stress management is an important part of most programmes of management (Levin *et al.* 1989).

Reaction times: practical issues

Given that reduced information processing rate is one of the basic effects of MHI (Levin *et al.* 1989, Lezac 1996), it is understandable that reaction times will be slower. Obviously this can put the patient at risk if they drive a car, use dangerous machinery, or engage in any activity where it

is important to be able to react quickly. Unfortunately, patients themselves will often be unaware that they are not responding normally.
Because their central nervous system clock has slowed down it seems
to them that they are reacting at the same speed as they have always
done. Thus it is important that they should have an objective assessment
of their ability to respond quickly before they are cleared to return to
activities where fast reaction times are needed.

It is also important that family and caregivers are told that the patient
should not drive their car or ride their motorbike until they have been
checked, as they will need to be the 'gatekeepers'. Occasionally the patient
may not want to accept this restriction. Usually they can be persuaded to
agree to leave the decision until there has been an on-road assessment
with an instructor who is experienced in the problems that people can
have after a head injury. It is not acceptable that they should be cleared
to drive on their own assessment alone.

People who have been injured at sport form a special subgroup of MHI
cases who need excellent reaction times before they return to their game,
and this issue is discussed fully in Chapter 12. Again it is important to
note that they will be poor judges of their own reaction times and independent assessment is needed.

Executive skills, planning, organizing, and monitoring

Imaging and neuropathological studies frequently show the frontal and
prefrontal areas to be affected in mild head injury. This is consistent with
the accounts of impaired executive function in these cases (Levin *et al.*
1989, Lezac 1996). The complaints will be that they cannot get motivated
to get started in an activity and cannot carry it through. For example,
they may realize that the lawn needs mowing and decide to do it 'soon',
but have a cup of coffee first, and then it becomes lunchtime; so the day
goes on. They may actually start to go to the shed to get the mower out
and then realize that it is pouring with rain. Meal preparation is particularly vulnerable to the effects of poor planning and organizing, as each
element needs to be prepared and cooked to be ready for eating at
the same time as the other parts of the meal. In this way, in the early
stages, the patient can get to the end of the day without ever having
achieved any of the goals that were set. Obviously, impaired executive
function will be as disabling as the effect of reduced information processing, which we have just described. It is also important to be aware
that it may not be obvious in the relatively structured environment of
the clinical interview.

Someone who has a demanding occupation or who sets high standards
for themselves will be more handicapped by impaired frontal lobe function than someone who is content to follow directions and only do as
much as they have to. Thus people who are high achievers will need to

recover more fully from these deficits before they are ready to return to work or to school.

Emotional lability

Emotional lability and mood swings are common after MHI and, like the problems with executive skills, probably result from impaired frontal lobe function. Typically they manifest themselves as an inappropriate over-reaction to rather trivial events. As with other behaviour problems there is a clear relation between the amount of self-control the patient can exert and the presence of fatigue and tension. Like the problems with executive function the mood swings, temper tantrums, or outbursts of tears often described as a 'personality change' are difficult for family to cope with and may lead to damaging problems with relationships.

Memory for words, faces, and places

To memorize anything we need to be able to attend to it (Lezac 1996). The ability to store and retrieve information therefore depends on the integrity of attention; in common with other areas of cognition it will vary with the level of fatigue and anxiety. Lezac has stressed this and pointed out that many so-called 'memory problems' are secondary to other deficits in basic functions. In essence, in most cases of mild head injury the ability to remember is intact, and memory function is compromised mainly because of reduced information processing capacity, abnormal fatigue, and secondary anxiety factors. This emphasizes the importance of getting a complete assessment before starting any treatment directed towards limited areas of deficit.

For the discussion at this stage we will examine the rare case where there is adequate ability to concentrate and where fatigue and stress are not major issues. Even in this case 'memory' is not a single unitary function. There can be interruption in the ability to place information into memory storage, so that the person has difficulty in learning new material; alternatively there may be difficulty in recalling this material later. These two different types of memory deficit are classified as problems with acquisition or retrieval; they can be combined in various proportions, and occasionally there is difficulty with both components. Significant deficits of this type are relatively rare after MHI, however, and probably reflect localized injury, particularly to hippocampal areas.

Modality specific memory problems also occur, probably reflecting both the diffuse information processing deficit together with more localized injury. For example, some patients may only have problems when they are trying to remember verbal material, others when the information is primarily visual or spatial. Thus verbal labels, particularly names of people, may be forgotten. Alternatively it may be difficult to recognize faces, or people may get lost even when they are trying to negotiate familiar routes. Usually there is some evidence of dysphasia in the first example, typically with focal damage in the left temporal or frontal area, and in the other two cases damage in the non-dominant hemisphere.

Visuo-spatial skills, judging distance, size, and shape

Deficits in these skills are important, even though they can be subtle, as they affect the ability to move about safely and interact with the environment. Thus it is common for patients to misjudge the position of an open door and collide with the frame or hit their head on a shelf because they have misjudged its height. Similarly the speed and location of traffic on the road may be misjudged and driving should not be allowed until it is clear that there has been recovery; pedestrians should also be warned of the need to take special care.

When these problems occur after mild injury it is rare for it to be possible to demonstrate localized lesions where they would be expected in the right temporal or parietal lobes, though presumably there is some pathology in these areas. Information processing ability is usually reduced and will be expected to interact with the specific deficits.

Understanding and using language

Problems with finding words, with following conversations, and with anticipating the end of a sentence are frequent complaints after MHI. As with the deficits described above they depend more on defective processing rather than localized damage to the frontal or temporal areas. Generally therefore they improve as the ability to concentrate improves, as focused attention is regained and distraction can be ignored.

Assessing cognitive function after mild head injury

The literature on mild head injury is heavily weighted towards descriptions of assessment techniques and test results, with a general consensus both about the types of behavioural and cognitive deficits that occur and about the time course of their recovery. We recommend the recent article by King (1997) as an excellent review. The non-specialist clinician for whom we have written this book will not always have the resources or staff with the expertise to assess for themselves or to carry out all the tests recommended in research reports. In this section we suggest how to make the best use of resources that are likely to be available, and how to decide when further investigations are needed.

Assessment – historical perspective

We have already described how, until the 1970s, persisting problems after mild head injury tended to be viewed as malingering or compensation neurosis, or both. This was to a large extent because assessments done by psychologists of the time were usually restricted to the standard Wechsler intelligence tests. Since they found no reduction of IQ they concluded that there had not been any after-effect of the injury. Further, there seemed to be only limited interest in enquiring why these patients continued to complain of a consistent and typical set of cognitive and behavioural effects, despite these negative results. Much of the reason may be that neuropsychology at that time was heavily influenced by the model which had been developed in Montréal after the war, which was concerned with the use of psychological tests to localize cerebral lesions. Closed head injury, particularly minor injury, could not fit within this model because at the time there was neither evidence of cerebral damage nor any method of anatomical localization.

There had been some earlier research reports of groups of head-injured cases which were compared with control groups on tests other than composite IQ measures, in particular on reaction time and attention tasks. However, it was not until the early 1970s that the clinical problem was specifically addressed and usable assessment techniques were developed (Levin *et al.* 1989). The time was ripe for a change for a number of reasons. Neuropsychology had progressed to something of a dead end with the pursuit of localization. Immense changes in imaging techniques, in particular the CT scan, could now show the position of a tumour or haemorrhage and there was less need to make a 'once removed' deduction on the basis of performance in a cognitive test. The contribution of neuropsychology to neurosurgery and neurology became the analysis and identification of the *effect* of the lesion rather than its *localization*. With this model, closed head injury, together with other conditions resulting in diffuse damage to the central nervous system, became a legitimate area of investigation.

At first the only objective evidence to suggest that there was an 'organic' effect of mild head injury came from neuropsychology, in particular from the demonstration of its effect on information processing ability. There remained, however, a considerable body of opinion which held that post-concussion problems were primarily psychological (Levin *et al.* 1989). Later, with the development of MR and SPECT procedures, there was definite evidence to support the view that they had indeed an organic basis. It is now generally accepted that the post-concussion syndrome has its basis in a mixture of the primary organic effects of the injury and the secondary psychological reactions to them.

General principles of assessment

There are some basic rules which apply whenever a head injury assessment is done. The first is that of *flexibility*. A set battery of tests which is administered in every case, regardless of status or performance during the session is a misuse of the examiner's time and of the patient's energy. It is pointless to give the patient every verbal memory test you have in your office if you have already found that they cannot learn a list of 15 words after the standard number of trials. The second rule is that of the *negative hypothesis*. That is that a negative result, in other words a normal performance on a particular test, does not mean that they have no problems with whatever cognitive function you assume the test measures. All it means is that you have not found any deficit on that test. By giving tests of increasing complexity you can increase the probability that any statement you make about the function is accurate, but even if they do well on every test you still cannot conclude that they have no deficit in that area. All the results mean is that you did not find any deficit during that session.

There are several factors to be taken into account in planning the timing and content of the assessment of a patient after a mild head injury, and these can be grouped into *injury* factors and *individual* factors.

Injury factors

Time since injury

It is quite uninformative to carry out an assessment in the first week after injury, since deficits in information processing ability, for example, are expected during this period and there will be no indication whether these will persist and with what degree of severity. On the other hand, an assessment done for the first time three or four months after the injury will probably be confounded by stress and anxiety factors and give a less straightforward picture of the organic basis of any problems. The ideal time for assessment is towards the end of the first month following the accident, when most patients have begun to make some functional recovery from the organic damage and before psychological factors have developed. At this stage it should be possible to identify the patients who are going to make up the 5–10 per cent who do not have an uneventful recovery, and so to begin appropriate interventions.

Unfortunately many patients are not referred until much later, in some cases at a year or even several years after the injury. Though it is unrealistic to expect a rapid or substantial improvement in a patient who has suffered from a full-blown post-concussion syndrome for this length of time, it is still important to document the cognitive and behavioural status of these people. This is so whether limited resources mean that all that can be offered is to give them some instruction on how to cope with their problems themselves, or whether intensive (and expensive) one-to-one work is begun to try to deal with the deficits.

Type of injury

It is important to document the details of the injury and the patient's condition at this time, together with the medical assessment of its severity.

When there has been a definite loss of consciousness the first assumption will be that any deficits found will be the result of the head injury. After whiplash and similar injuries, where there has been no loss of consciousness, symptoms of the post-concussion type may be the presenting problem, but it may be necessary to produce special evidence that the injury described was the cause. The assessment in this case has to be particularly thorough, both to confirm that the deficits are typical of the PCS and to exclude other causes.

The composition of the assessment also depends on other injuries that were sustained in the accident. Trivial examples are that if the dominant arm was injured, tests needing a written response cannot be used, and that the battery will have to be modified if sight or hearing has been affected. Assessment will be unreliable if other injuries are causing pain and fatigue, or if strong analgesics are being used. If the patient is immobilized and unable to return to work or school it will not be appropriate to make a full assessment, at least in the earlier weeks.

Stage of recovery

Headache and fatigue are likely to be problems with any patients recommended for assessment and these will affect the composition and duration of any session. As a general guideline it is usually the case that in the first month after the injury the patient will be unable to tolerate more than 30 minutes at a time. Though this limits the scope of the initial testing, it does ensure that the results indicate the optimum level of performance without reduction due to fatigue. Even after the early period, this basic principle of assessment needs to apply. The fatigue level and physical state of the patient must determine when the session has to be ended and when it can be resumed. Similar constraints apply to the time of day when the assessment is made. Sleep cycles are often disturbed after MHI and appointments should avoid times when the patient would usually be tired or having a sleep.

Individual factors

Premorbid level of ability

Evaluation of cognitive data is most straightforward when the subject falls within the average 85 per cent of the population, since most comparison data have been developed for this 'normal' group. There are various methods of estimating premorbid ability and of deciding whether the 'normal' control data are appropriate. Obviously some people fall above or below this level and it is important that they are not disadvantaged by an assessment designed for people who were less or more able than they had been before their injury.

The above-average patient is particularly at risk, in that a superficial assessment may conclude they are not impaired in any cognitive domain, because they scored at an average level on all measures. In fact for them an average level of performance may represent a significant deficit. The battery of tests therefore needs to include both demanding measures and those that are less affected by IQ and education.

Low-functioning patients can also be disadvantaged, since it may be difficult to establish whether a low score is the result of the head injury. This is likely to have been the cause if scores on some measures are significantly lower than on others. This is of limited value, however, as many measures used in the assessment of the general population have a 'floor' effect, where there is a level below which the scores are unable to discriminate between different poor performers. This may result when the task is too difficult for any of the lower scorers to achieve, which might occur, for example, if it was a difficult calculation (there can also be a 'ceiling' effect, when the task is an easy one such as reciting the alphabet, when the mean score will be close to the maximum).

Occupation and employment status

The degree to which cognitive deficits will affect the patient's ability to function will depend on their occupation and employment, and the composition of the test battery must take this into account. As an example a student must have good powers of concentration to enable them to read their texts and to take in lecturers, and a competent memory to retain what they have read and been taught. A cabinet maker has somewhat different needs, and a long distance truck driver others. All need to be able to manage fatigue and to control mood swings and irritability. The assessment must take all of these factors into account.

If the patient is unemployed they still need an appropriate assessment. It is sometimes held that they have fewer demands to meet and therefore fewer problems, but this is not so for two main reasons. The first is that if they are looking for work, and this is the usual situation, it is necessary to know their strengths and weaknesses so that they can be guided into an area where they have the best chance of succeeding; rehabilitation which is vocationally relevant can then be planned. The other reason is that the minority who have no motivation to work are at risk of focusing on post-concussion symptoms rather than actual deficits, and of using them to prolong their 'sickness'. Good grounds are needed if the rehabilitation staff are going to insist that they can get back to the work force if they really try and that they have to behave sensibly and avoid fatigue, alcohol, and drugs.

The 'ideal' assessment

This section describes the procedures which are important in an examination of the cognitive and behavioural effects of a mild head injury. The members of the management team principally involved will be the neuropsychologist and the clinical psychologist. An occupational therapist will be included if there are other injuries which affect the activities of daily living; they need to be familiar with the effects of fatigue and impaired attention in MHI. A speech and language therapist will be able to contribute when it is necessary to distinguish between deficits due to specific local damage and the effects of generalized head injury.

In an ideal situation, where cost was not an issue, anyone who sustained a mild head injury would be assessed by such a team three or four weeks after the accident, so that if there were significant defects their return to work or school could be managed.

The neuropsychologist's assessment

A full neuropsychological assessment can take several sessions to administer, and this is neither practical nor appropriate in the great majority of patients with a mild head injury. The constraints on session time and the selection of tests are commented on earlier in this chapter. In the present section we will give a brief outline of the families of tests available to the neuropsychologist and give some guidelines on deciding which to use, depending on the needs of the particular patient. As noted above, we do not advise that a set battery of tests should be used for all cases, but recommend that the assessment be flexible, adding or omitting tasks depending on performance and circumstances. Nor will we attempt to give a menu of specific tests or describe the details of administration, since this information is readily available to all psychologists (see, for example, Lezac 1996, Spleen and Strauss 1997). However, to illustrate each area we refer to some of the tests included in the MHI assessments in our clinic, and give our personal preferences. It is important to stress, though, that not all neuropsychologists would use these specific tests, nor is it necessary that they do so.

Two types of information will be provided by this assessment. The first is the *quantitative data*, which will consist of the actual test score, giving a measure of how well the patient coped with the task compared to other people in the range of ability and age specified in the control data. This measure is most useful for people who fell within the average range before the injury, but is only a general guide for people whose premorbid ability was above or below the average.

The second type of information is *qualitative*. This refers to the observations gathered during the session of how the patient attacked each task, whether they became distracted by extraneous noise, whether their concentration varied over time, whether they tired quickly or became restless, and so on. So that they can make these observations most clinical neuropsychologists prefer to administer the tests themselves, rather than handing them over to a psychometrician, as they are aware that the qualitative data are equally as important as the quantitative data.

Tests available

Tests of premorbid ability   Several tests of this family are available. Most of them are relatively quick to administer, important because even the shortest test session needs to include some estimate of premorbid ability. The New Adult Reading Test (NART) meets the criteria of brevity and reliability. The NART has a list of words to read with all of them having spelling that does not help with pronunciation (e.g. 'ache'). The rationale is that if the word has been in the reader's vocabulary before the illness or injury, pronunciation would not be impaired even if the ability to define the word had been lost.

Tests of orientation in time and place and *tests of the continued presence of post-traumatic amnesia*   We have found the Westmead PTA scale more useful than the Galveston Orientation and Amnesia Test (GOAT) which has no objective measure of memory function. However, neither is sufficiently discriminative for MHI cases, where the duration of PTA is likely to be less than 24 h. The Westmead, for instance, defines the end of the period of PTA as the first of three consecutive days when all the questions are answered correctly.

These tests are only needed if the patient is being examined in the period immediately after the accident. Note that some patients may be disorientated and not amnesic, and vice versa.

Tests of attention and concentration   Every assessment should include some measures of attention, and in particular tests which provide an estimate of information processing capacity. These can vary from brief tasks to difficult and demanding ones which would not be appropriate for all cases. The Paced Auditory Serial Addition Test (PASAT) is such a task. This was selected specifically because it is sensitive to attention impairment after MHI. There are four trials, presented at increasingly fast rates, and in high functioning individuals it is usually the two fastest rates that are the most useful in detecting mild impairment. The original protocol for PASAT has had many changes made by other workers, including shortening trial length, increasing the interstimulus interval so that it can be used with severely head-injured cases, and using only the two slowest pacing rates, which obviously reduces its usefulness for MHI cases. We have also had to make changes, but not in the structure or administration. It has given us important information about how MHI patients function, and we still use a taped version produced from a master copy made 20 years ago. However, when we first reported PASAT results we cited correlation coefficients obtained by Sampson in the 1950s (Sampson 1954) using a large sample of service personnel. These showed only minimal correlation between PASAT performance and arithmetic ability or general intelligence. More recent work has found significant correlations between both. In some studies this was probably because the versions of PASAT that were used differed from that originally used by Sampson. However, there is now convincing evidence from an excellent recent paper by Crawford *et al.* (1998) using the same procedure as we do, that while PASAT loads highly on the Wechsler Adult Intelligence Scale, Revised (WAIS-R) attention/concentration factor, there was an almost equally high loading on general intelligence. Crawford's subject sample was drawn from the general public, and thus from a more heterogeneous group than that used by Sampson, which no doubt accounts for the difference between the two sets of correlations. In any case the Crawford data are more compelling, since their subjects were more representative of the population of MHI cases.

We also usually include some subtests from the Thames Tests of Everyday Attention (TEA). These are brief and based on everyday skills, so that they have a higher face validity than a test such as PASAT. We have also found them useful in cases where English is not the first language, though we do not as yet have adequate normative data. The four subtests we use most frequently are the Map test, when the subject must circle as many target symbols as they can find on a complex map of the Philadelphia area in a 2 minute period; the Telephone task, where they have to circle all paired symbols on a large sheet designed to look like listings for restaurants in the *Yellow Pages*; a dual task in which they have to do the same Telephone test on another sheet (this time with hotels) at the same time as counting strings of tones presented on a tap; and the Lottery test, a vigilance type task in which they have to listen for infrequent target stimuli over an extended period.

If the patient has only a limited tolerance of fatigue the rule should be to begin with a simple test, and only move to more complex tests if they cope with the easier ones. Note that as we mentioned above the qualitative information that you record during the session will also provide valuable information about concentration span and the ability to ignore distraction.

Tests of reaction time   Every assessment should include a test of reaction time, unless the patient's condition, such as immobilization by other injuries or constant pain, makes it impractical. Simple reaction time tests measure the time it takes to make a given response (e.g. a key press) to a given signal (e.g. a tone or light). The only decision making that is needed is a yes−no one, that is, that the signal has or has not been given. This contrasts with complex reaction time tests where one of several responses must be made, depending on which of a number of signals has been given. Both can be equally sensitive to slowing in the patient with a severe head injury, but most studies show that complex reaction time tasks are more sensitive in detecting the effects of MHI. The tests most often used give an estimate of response times to visual stimuli. They should involve the peripheral as well as the central fields and be able to compare the responses to stimuli on the left and right as well as at the centre of the field. We have gathered an extensive amount of control data on the Compreact test and we use this more than any other.

Tests of frontal lobe function   Composite tasks where planning and organizational skills can be assessed are useful here. It is important only to use tests that have been well established as reliable and valid measures, as not all are acceptable. Because most of these tasks are complex and multifactorial in nature, performance can be impaired for reasons other than impaired executive skills. Thus we rarely use the Wisconsin Card Sorting Test, though it has a long history as a test of frontal lobe function, partly because of the large number of false positives and false negatives that have been reported, and partly because high functioning individuals can do poorly because they attempt to use complicated rules for sorting instead of the basic colour, shape, and number categories. Similarly the Tower of London task (or Tower of Hanoi), where the object is to work out a system for moving different sized pieces from one pile to another, is both not always able to discriminate even severely head-injured subjects from controls, but also can be failed for many reasons other than impaired planning and organizational skills. We are aware that the same reservations apply to the three measures we use most frequently, the controlled word fluency test, the WAIS-R block design subtest, and the copy trial of the Rey-Osterreith complex figure. Obviously visual perceptual problems can impair performance on the latter two, and language deficits or limited vocabulary can affect word fluency. Thus the qualitative information, how the patient approaches each task during the session, is equally important, and it is the combination of the two types of evidence, plus the history from the family and the patient, that allows one to arrive at a decision.

Tests of general intelligence   Most psychologists include a standard intelligence test in their repertoire. The most widely used are the Wechsler tests, consisting of numerous subtests. These typically take several hours to administer. There is no reason to give the full set of subtests, at least until three or four months after the accident, but useful information can be gained from selected ones. Even if all the subtests are given, they should not be used to provide an IQ score. Deficits in response speed and concentration, or in abstract reasoning may be lost within a composite score, and the IQ itself is meaningless if it is confounded by one or several deviant scores.

Tests of memory All assessments need to include measures of verbal and non-verbal memory, of the ability to recall information immediately and after a delay period. They need to examine the ability to recall information and recognize it when it is presented in a set of statements that the patient has not previously seen or heard. There are also many other parameters to memory tasks such as complexity and difficulty. Given that memory function varies and depends on a person's IQ, it is clearly important to select tests that are appropriate to the patient's premorbid ability. In addition, memory, of all the areas of cognitive function, is the domain where it is most important to take into account the other effects of the injury and the individual factors we mentioned above. No one will have an effective memory if they are tired or have a headache, and no one who has had learning problems at school will do well in a memory test after a head injury.

The Selective Reminding Test has been used since the 1970s to assess verbal learning in both adults and children, and thus there is a good body of background evidence in the literature. We used to give this to most patients, but as more and more accounts of Rey Auditory Verbal Learning Test (RAVLT) performance in cases of MHI have been reported this is now our main test. It allows an estimate of acquisition, performance after distraction, and delay and also recognition memory for the information. The Wechsler prose passages, with both immediate and delayed recall, are used to assess memory for narrative material. We also find that the incidental learning measure from the WAIS-RNI digit symbol subtest gives useful information about memory function. To assess non-verbal memory we have used the visual sequential memory (VSM) subtest from the Illinois Test of Psycholinguistic Ability (ITPA). Although the ITPA is a test designed for children under 10 years old, we found that VSM is appropriate even for high functioning university students, since the sampling procedure means that people can be tested at their own level, and since it has a high enough ceiling to ensure that it is very rare for adults to score 100 per cent. The other measure of non-verbal memory we use is the 30 minute recall trial of the Rey complex figure. However, results on this will be confounded if the person had difficulty even when they had the figure in front of them to copy.

Test of visual perception and visuo-motor skills Tests such as the Rey–Osterreith complex figure, which include both immediate and delayed recall of visual information, give the most efficient use of session time. It is also sensible to include visuo-constructional tasks, since they are able to provide a structured situation for testing executive functions.

Tests of language function   In the case of a mild head injured patient it is not generally necessary to administer a full battery of expressive and receptive language tests. Careful observation during the session will usually detect problems with naming or word finding. In the acute period, three or four weeks after the injury, it is better to concentrate on the other domains, which will be the most important ones for the assessment of their needs. In the longer term, if language difficulties persist, it is more appropriate to involve the speech–language therapists to identify the areas of deficit.

The clinical psychologist's assessment

The contribution of the clinical psychologist to the assessment is to evaluate emotional status, check for the presence and degree of depression, and to examine the patient's reaction to the trauma of the injury. As well as an in-depth interview, this will include the use of specially designed questionnaires and rating scales. Family and social issues will be examined in some detail, as these factors will need to be taken into account in planning the management of recovery, and also be relevant in interpreting the results of the neuropsychological assessment.

The clinical psychologist has a special role in establishing the contribution of post-traumatic stress disorder (PTSD). This is discussed in more detail in Chapter 11.

Follow-up assessments

Regular reassessment of the patient is important, for two reasons: the first being to monitor their performance and adjust the demands that their programme makes on them. The second is to give them objective information on the progress they are making. The frequency of the assessments will vary with the time since the accident. Changes occur most rapidly in the first six months, and to begin with the patient should be seen every two weeks until a stable pattern of improvement is seen. Three-monthly assessments will then usually be adequate, with special sessions if there are signs that recovery is not going smoothly for any reason, or if the time has come for a trial of return to work.

At a reassessment there is seldom any need to repeat the entire set of tests that was administered at the first session. Obviously, areas where there had been deficits need to be checked again. The usual caveats about practice effects must of course be taken into account. Either parallel forms of the test should be used if they are available, or tests with known practice effects (e.g. PASAT) should be used. The neuropsychologist working in the team should therefore have a supply of alternative measures to cover the needs of multiple reassessments.

Practical compromises

Few health systems are able to provide a comprehensive assessment and management programme such as we have described for every person who has a mild head injury. Further, because most patients will make an uneventful recovery (Ruff *et al.* 1993), it would be a waste of time, both for the system and for the patient. However, even where there is some recognition of the advantages of screening those with a higher chance of persistent problems, only a few areas are likely to provide the facilities and expert staff which can carry out a comprehensive assessment such as we have described. These problems are discussed in Chapter 9.

One solution is to establish satellite clinics in smaller towns outside the major cities, with regular visits from the central clinic staff who can provide advice and monitor the service. Most towns will have at least one clinical psychologist in the area who would be capable of carrying out screening assessments with the support of the clinical neuropsychologist from the main clinic. Provided that some postgraduate training was available for those who had not worked with people with mild head injuries, they would be capable of checking mood changes and other responses to trauma.

The patient and their family as informants

Essential to management is the information that is provided by the patient and their family. As time goes by they are in the best position to know if there has been any deterioration in behaviour or cognition, and their reports give valuable pointers to the areas which it is important to examine and assess. The lack of insight and denial of impairment that is common in patients with a more severe injury is rare after MHI, and whilst the patient may not volunteer information about negative behaviour such as aggression and irritability, the family will certainly do so, out of concern to get advice and help.

It is particularly useful to listen to the comments of someone who was functioning at a comparatively high level before the injury. Their performance on memory tests may show average scores, but they may tell you that they cannot do things as quickly or as efficiently as before. A good history from the family will be important in confirming that the patient's account of poor performance is accurate. Again, if it is established that they used to manage a busy office, juggle several different queries at once, and never needed to use a diary, but now can't cope with even half a day's work, this will be of more significance than an average score in a quiet test room with no distractions.

However, a condition termed the 'halo' effect, found in families with a member who has a severe head injury, does sometimes occur after a mild head injury. The relief that their family member has survived after a dramatic accident may blind them to faults that were certainly present beforehand. Thus there can be a tendency to blame the injury for any failure, of memory or behaviour, forgetting what used to happen before.

Malingering

If someone complains that they continue to have disabling problems after a mild head injury, the only evidence, apart from their account of their symptoms, is the cognitive and behavioural assessment we have described. At present neither electrodiagnostic tests, MR nor SPECT, can offer useful support. The cognitive data have tended to be regarded as 'soft', since to accept them the clinician has to believe that the patient has not been exaggerating their subjective complaints or cheating in the neuropsychological tests.

The DSM-III-R definition has not made it easier to sort out the issue, as it proposes that in malingerers there is a disparity between subjective complaints and objective evidence, that they mostly expect some financial gain from presenting with disability, and that they may have been engaged in antisocial behaviour. These are all conditions that are met by people with genuine post-concussion problems as well as by malingerers.

It is not surprising therefore that there has been considerable effort spent on methods of distinguishing between those who have genuine problems and those who are attempting to 'defraud the system'. This has come about largely as a result of the vast litigation industry, particularly in North America. There are numerous reports of tests which have been shown to differentiate between groups known to have persisting problems after mild head injury and others who have been instructed to perform on the tests as though they had been injured. Most of the tests have been of memory, and have been based on the premise that the malingerer is likely to do badly on all tests, even those that are not generally sensitive to head injury, and that they will score even below the level that would be expected if responding was by chance. There have also been attempts to devise statistical formulae that can be applied to sets of test results to determine whether they can be accepted as genuine. A comprehensive selection of these tests can be found in Lezak's *Neuropsychological assessment* (1996).

It has been our experience that frank malingering is rare in our population, perhaps because of the no-fault compensation system in New Zealand. This section, therefore, draws heavily on writers who work elsewhere. In particular we have relied on the excellent account published by Ruff *et al.* in 1993. They cite Resnick's conclusion that it is not possible to make a definite diagnosis unless there has been an actual confession from the malingerer, or if they had been seen carrying out activities that they had claimed that for them were impossible. They also point out the ethical and practical consequences of incorrectly classifying symptoms or test results as malingered. They advise that an integrated approach needs to be used if malingering is suspected, with 'seasoned clinicians' comparing both the objective and subjective data. More specific tests they list are the following.

(1) Reassess the patient to see if the same results are obtained.

(2) Review premorbid school and medical records.

(3) Interview family and friends, and the patient, to get a good idea of premorbid as well as post-morbid function.

(4) Find out what financial gain the patient could expect and how vital this would be to the patient.

(5) Look at the independence of data measures, since inconsistency on one measure does not allow one to conclude that all other test responses are flawed.

In our clinic we have found that to many people head injury has negative implications, and that they tend to put head injury, intellectual handicap, and psychiatric illness into the same category. MHI patients do not want to be in this category, or to be thought to be impaired in this way. It is more common for these people to expend an abnormal effort to produce a 'normal' score, even if this leaves them so fatigued that they fall asleep once they have left the test room. When the opposite occurs, and a poorer than possible performance suggests that the patient is deliberately faking, this often seems to be a cry for help. The patient is aware of the myriad of changes that have occurred since the injury, but perhaps every medical examination has told him or her that there is nothing wrong. However, the patient knows that he or she is forgetful, cannot concentrate, and tires easily, and so seizes the neuropsychological assessment as an opportunity to show someone that he or she does indeed have problems.

We have found that discussing the aberrant results with the patients, explaining why they are a concern, and also giving them assurance that we do accept that their problems exist is usually all that is needed. If, in addition, they are included in a formal programme where they are able to interact with other people and carry out various activities under supervision, it is possible to verify whether they are genuinely disabled by the injury. For example, if there is a young man who complains of continual headaches but who plays table tennis for as long as there are partners and takes part in a noisy discussion, it is most likely that they are exaggerating how bad their headaches are. Another young man who is unable to concentrate on a form he is filling out when there is any other activity in the room, and who cannot enjoy watching a video because he can't remember the characters or the plot, is likely to be genuine, even if his original assessment showed some discrepancies.

References

Crawford, J. R., Obonsawin, M. C., and Allan, K. M. (1998). PASAT and components of WAIS-R performance: convergent and discriminant validity. *Assessment of Attention and Executive Functions*, Special Issue: *Neuropsychological Rehabilitation*, **8**, pp. 255–72.

King, N. (1997) Mild Head Injury: neuropathology, sequelae, measurement and recovery. *British Journal of Clinical Psychology*, **36**, 161–84.

Levin, H. S., Eisenberg, H. M., and Benton, A. L. (eds) (1989). *Mild head injury.* Oxford University Press, New York.

Lezac, M. D. (1996). *Neuropsychological assessment*, (3rd ed). Oxford University Press, New York.

This is a classic textbook, widely used since its first edition 20 years ago.

Ruff, R. M., Wylie, T., and Woodrow, T. (1993). Malingering and malingering-like aspects of mild closed head injury. *Journal of Head Trauma Rehabilitation*, **8**, 60–73.

An excellent, relatively recent discussion of the malingering issue.

Sampson, H. (1954) Correlations between performance on serial addition tests and general and arithmetical ability, Unpublished research data cited in Gronwall, D. M. A. and Sampson, H. (1974) *The Psychological Effects of Concussion*, Oxford University Press, Auckland.

Spreen, O. and Strauss, E. (1997). *A compendium of neuropsychological tests. Administration, norms and commentary,* (2nd edn). Oxford University Press, New York.

A comprehensive compendium of tests which covers every area that may be needed for an MHI assessment; a useful 'cookbook' for experienced psychologists.

9
Principles of management

Introduction

In previous chapters we have looked at various aspects of the syndrome of mild head injury. In this section we will try to bring these together into a rational scheme for practical management.

We will start by mentioning the physiological basis of recovery and some factors which affect it. We will then discuss the first diagnosis and contact with the patient and their family and the establishment of a relationship with them. Setting up a programme for management follows, with a description of the various elements of the syndrome which need to be considered. Monitoring progress and the steps towards return to work are then discussed. Lastly we consider the organization of a service for people with mild head injury.

Factors in the recovery of function

In Chapter 3 we described the neuronal death, axonal injury, and changes in perfusion which can occur after mild head injury. Though there is evidence that there are some attempts at neuronal repair it seems unlikely that this is important in the recovery of function after injury. The dominant factor is more likely to be reprogramming of intact neuronal circuits and the use of the great reserve of these that the brain possesses. Presumably this is achieved by working repeatedly through the sort of situations that formed the original connections, both those of everyday living and of more complex intellectual tasks. This process will need the organization and executive capacity of the frontal lobes, and so will be less efficient if these have been damaged.

Recovery achieved in this way may be remarkable, but the fact remains that the mechanism has been damaged and capacity reduced. Though function may be adequate under normal conditions, when the patient is tired or stressed or has taken alcohol, or if they have a further head injury, performance will deteriorate.

Age is an important factor. In older people recovery is slower and is more likely to be incomplete, perhaps because the number of neurons available is smaller. Children learn more easily, but their development depends on an orderly time sequence and an injury may interrupt this and result in problems later.

Of the clinical factors adversely affecting recovery, the two most important are abnormal fatigue and the patient's reaction to their disability. These work together, with recovery being further impeded by the depression which so often follows.

Stages at which patients come for help

As we described in Chapter 5, patients who come for help fall into three general groups – early, middle, and late. In the early group, somatic symptoms are usually prominent, with fatigue and poor concentration. Those in the middle group complain of poor concentration and memory, inability to cope with work or study, fatigue, and irritability, and again some of the somatic symptoms. In the late group there has been a degree of disability for months or years, with fatigue and failure to perform up to expectation, and behavioural and family problems.

In Chapter 2 we saw that in the author's clinic about 25 per cent of the patients were likely to be in the acute phase, 60 per cent in the middle group, and 15 per cent in the late group.

Initial measures

The first step is to decide whether the clinical picture that the patient presents with is in fact due to the head injury described. In most cases the history and symptoms will leave the diagnosis in little doubt. Neurological and neuropsychological assessments will confirm it, and indicate areas where there are problems which need special attention.

Next, an estimate is needed of the part played by secondary symptoms, by anxiety, and family tensions. The financial situation should be explored, to determine what the resources of the family are, what insurance cover exists, and whether a legal action for damages is likely (see Chapter 13).

It is important that there should be contact with family – parents or spouse – from the first, both to expand and corroborate the patient's account and to explain what has happened and how they can help with management.

Difficulties in diagnosis

There may be uncertainty if there is an excessive or atypical reaction to an injury, which might suggest that there was either a pre-existing emotional instability or deliberate deception. The doubt will usually be resolved by the results of the neuropsychological tests, which in suspect cases are likely to show disproportion between the deficits and the symptoms; obvious inconsistencies within the tests may indicate frank malingering (see Chapter 8). However, even where the pattern of test results is that typically found after MHI, a history of instability or psychiatric illness may be used in litigation to deny liability.

Patients of the late group give rise to most difficulty in diagnosis. After the lapse of time the connection with the injury may be uncertain. The emotional reaction to a long-lasting unexplained disability may suggest that the symptoms were of psychiatric origin from the outset. If there is negotiation for compensation it may have been suspected that the symptoms are being exaggerated. In coming to a decision a well documented evidence of a change of capacity at work or in home-making clearly related to the accident will be important. most weight will be placed on the results of neuropsychological testing. A consistent deficit in one or more areas will support an organic origin. Sometimes it is difficult to be sure of the diagnosis, and the response to a trial rehabilitation programme may be helpful.

Explaining the situation

To some patients the cause of their symptoms will have been apparent all along. Others, perhaps when the effects appear to have been out of proportion to the severity of the injury, will often say that they thought they had a brain tumour or were going mad, and are enormously relieved when they understand the cause.

Having been told the diagnosis the patient and family will want to know what the future holds. Sometimes if the condition is either very mild or very severe it may be possible to give a definite answer. Usually it is best to say that it is just impossible to forecast until the response to treatment can be seen. After such a trial period it may be reasonable to give an estimate, but again it will be essential to say that not only is it impossible to put a definite time to recovery, but that to do so may be damaging if it raises expectations that are not met. This may be one of the most difficult things for patient and family to accept.

Setting up a programme

When the diagnosis has been made it will usually be the physician and the neuropsychologist who will plan the initial programme. Apart from treatment for particular medical conditions, the principal needs will be to deal with stress and fatigue and to set up a plan for activities that will give the patient a regular structured day. How this should be done must be explained to the patient and their family and ways and means discussed with them. Most patients will need outside help to get started on a programme, and continuing support to keep them going.

The minimum help, which may be enough in the mildest cases, is to explain to the patient carefully what the problems are and how to deal with them and to give them an information booklet to refer to. Follow-up visits every two or three weeks may be enough to check progress and deal with any difficulties.

Most patients will not be able to organize themselves sufficiently well without more help than this. They will need to see rehabilitation staff each week or even more often. If this involves travelling the extra burden may outweigh the benefit, and visiting staff may be needed to make the programme effective. When it is possible a period of residential treatment may be indicated. The practical problems of setting up a service to deal with these problems is discussed later in this chapter.

Sleep

In the early days after injury patients will usually sleep for longer hours, going to bed early and getting up late, and often needing an extra period of sleep during the day. Managing the sleep pattern is an important part of managing fatigue and it should be explained to them when they begin the programme that sufficient sleep is an essential key to a good recovery. Often they will be reluctant to 'give in' and have a sleep when they need it, pushing themselves to stay awake because 'only babies sleep in the afternoons'. Usually this can be overcome by giving them accurate feedback about the difference between how they function when they have rested and when they are tired.

As they improve they will gradually need less sleep. However, the pattern may change suddenly, usually with them having difficulty in getting to sleep and then waking every two or three hours and lying awake. This typically happens if they are under stress, either self-imposed because they have not fully recovered and are trying to do too much, or when there is financial, family, or work pressure. Sometimes it occurs when they have cut out their afternoon sleep and have become over-tired and hyperactive. In either case the first intervention should be relaxation training. At first this needs to be on a one-to-one basis to find out which technique is most effective for them. Once they have found a system which works in securing an adequate sleep pattern it is often useful to attend group 'refresher sessions' to maintain the improvement.

Not all patients respond to counselling and relaxation techniques, and for them medication may be appropriate (see Chapter 10).

Managing fatigue and stress

The first stage in managing the patient who is not recovering spontaneously from a mild head injury is to show them how to deal with both stress and fatigue, as these will limit how much they can do. Both must be well under control before significant improvement can be expected. A stress management programme should be incorporated early on, so that the patient can learn to recognize the early somatic signs and develop techniques to cope with stress before it becomes a major problem. Follow-up sessions should be held on a regular basis, and there should be a way of setting up crisis counselling if it is needed.

The next step is to explain to the patient the limitations that fatigue places on them and to identify the activities that they find particularly tiring. They will probably have noticed that since the accident every activity that involves concentration and mental activity affects them in this way, and it is important to explain that this is to be expected after the injuries that they have had. They need to be reassured that their ability to tolerate fatigue will increase as they recover.

It is necessary to establish how much the patient can do before they feel tired. This will be based partly on careful observations during the assessment sessions, and partly from their own account, and that of their family, of what they are actually able to achieve when they are at home. Based on this a daily schedule can be set up, with rest or sleep periods as needed, putting the most demanding activities in the morning when they are most alert.

Family and rehabilitation staff will need to monitor this schedule, adjusting it on the basis of actual performance and encouraging the patient to rest when it becomes plain that they are coming close to reaching their limit. To begin with the patient will be a poor judge of how tired they are, but an observer will notice that their attention has become erratic, and perhaps they are pale or their eyes look glazed. In addition they are likely to become irritable and less tolerant of noise. The aim should be for patients themselves to learn to recognize the symptoms in their early stage, to stop whatever they are doing before the fatigue becomes established, and to make sensible use of rest or sleep periods during the day.

When the patient has settled into a routine in which they have control of their fatigue, the schedule can be built up gradually, still with careful monitoring and taking account of special events such as unexpected visitors or family occasions. As they improve, they may find that they are able to cope with short and untaxing jobs around the home, and eventually an hour or two a day at their usual work. It is important that they demonstrate that they are able to cope with each stage before moving on to the next.

As well as the patient's own report and the observations of the rehabilitation staff, progress should be monitored on a regular basis with neuropsychological tests, so that any changes can be responded to promptly and the programme can be modified if there has been no improvement. Clearly this assessment is particularly important when a major change is contemplated, such as beginning part-time work.

However well monitored it may be, the situation is fragile, particularly in the later stages when the patient is in the process of getting back to their normal work. It may be that when they have finished the hours of work that have been agreed on they feel fine and decide to go ahead and finish the job. Perhaps their conscience pushes them, or their workmates, their employer, or the bank manager, seeing someone who looks physically fit, tell them that they can do that extra piece of work if they really try. They battle on, and become overtired. That evening, symptoms they have not had for some time come back. They start the next day without clearing their fatigue completely, have to struggle to achieve their target, and end the day with an even greater debt of fatigue. After a day or two they are too exhausted to continue and need to take substantial time off to recover. This 'boom or bust' cycle has to be avoided. It results in feelings of guilt and failure, which adds to their stress and depression and further diminishes their capacity.

The situation and the possibilities must be clearly explained to the patient and they must understand them and contract to accept responsibility for staying within the agreed levels of activity. However, even with the most reliable patient, the situation can still be unstable, and difficulties at work, family problems, or a heavy social weekend can set them back. It may be necessary to reduce working hours for a time or even to have a few days of complete rest to put things right.

Managing reduced ability to attend and concentrate

In most cases difficulty with attention and concentration should be managed by showing the patient how to deal with fatigue and stress. Situations in which there is too much information to deal with must be avoided. Complex activities have to be broken down into simpler components which do not exceed the available information processing capacity.

Managing structure

Executive functions are very commonly impaired after MHI. Patients find it difficult to plan and organize their day, then find that they cannot keep to task, get distracted, and end up not actually completing anything that they had planned to do. They need help in setting up a structured day. This needs to be more than directions to 'make lists' and to 'set goals'. These instructions tend to result either in an unrealistic set of tasks which will make impossible demands on their ability to cope without fatigue, or an unrealistically complex activity such as 'tidy workshop', which results in inertia where they don't even know where to start.

Rehabilitation staff need to work out with the patient and the family what are the reasonable goals for a day, considering the stage of recovery and the fatigue tolerance. Each activity needs to be broken down into simple steps, and written out in list form in consecutive order for the patient to check off as they are completed. It is important to incorporate this structure within the fatigue management programme and to have the list on a permanent visible structure such as a whiteboard, or in a notebook which the patient can carry in their pocket if necessary. An electronic aid such as hourly alarms on a wrist watch can be used as a reminder to check the list.

Management of memory and other cognitive problems

We have found that usually the biggest hurdle in overcoming memory deficits is the patient's determination not to use diaries and other memory aids, because they never needed them before their accident and they want their memory to be as good as it was then. Counselling and support from other patients who have gone through similar stages is often useful in getting over this hurdle. If they can be reassured that the best way of overcoming the problem is to take the load off their memory by writing things down they can usually be persuaded to try a diary, calendar, or electronic aid. We explain that if you reduce the stress and concern that an important event or piece of information will be forgotten, the probability of remembering it is increased.

In those cases where a specific memory deficit remains after other abilities have recovered, the gamut of memory remediation techniques that are available can be tried. In our clinic, however, we have found it more effective and cheaper to set up simple or perhaps electronic systems to compensate for the problems.

Managing behaviour problems

Irritability, anger, and loss of self-control are destructive to the patient's rehabilitation as well as to their family and friendships. Counselling that the patient has received in the techniques of stress management should help them to avoid conflict, to recognize when they are becoming irritated and worked up, and teach them to take time out away from the situation. Practical measures will help, such as turning down loud music or asking another family to have the children to play. If these measures are not effective, medication, perhaps with carbamazepine, may be useful (see Chapter 10). More elaborate psychotherapy is rarely needed.

Physical condition

The change of lifestyle which occurs when a patient is recovering from a head injury will usually reduce the amount of physical activity and formal exercise they take, and the loss of condition that follows may slow their recovery. As soon as possible they should start whatever gentle exercise they can manage, the limitation usually being headache, and they should increase this as they improve.

Counselling and support

Patients will need the opportunity for extended contact and discussion with rehabilitation staff to help them with the problems that are described above. As well as this help should be available from specialist counsellors if the secondary effects of disability are severe.

The patient has to deal with the general unpleasantness of physical symptoms such as headache and dizziness, and with the restriction of their usual pleasures and the things which make them feel good – family and social life, work, hobbies, and sports. They tend to lose contact with the people they are accustomed to meeting every day, who often find it difficult to understand how someone with no visible evidence of something wrong can be so disabled. They generally have financial difficulties, with meeting bills and with rent or mortgage payments. Almost all have at least some of these problems, and it is not surprising that many of them become significantly depressed.

It is important that counselling and support are in place as soon as it seems that disability is likely to last for more than a short time. The patient should be reassured that their problems are both understood and understandable. Family and friends should be put into the picture, and if reasonable, workmates and employer too. Having information sheets and booklets available will help with this.

Relations between partners can become strained. The uninjured partner may have to take on extra responsibilities for children, other household tasks, and perhaps the maintenance of an income. Loss of sexual activity may be difficult to cope with. Before they become serious and irreversible these problems should be dealt with by an experienced family counsellor who is familiar with the special problems arising from MHI.

A source of financial advice should be available, as should the means of putting patients in touch with lawyers expert in handling disability claims (see Chapter 13). Patients will vary greatly in the extent to which they choose to make use of help of this sort, but expert and appropriate counselling must always be available and offered when it seems to be needed.

As well as professional counselling, support groups of current and old patients can be valuable. Indeed, often a valuable therapist for someone with an MHI will be another MHI patient. They can realize that they are not alone and can learn how others have dealt with the problems they have now. It is, however, best that there should be an experienced professional counsellor present at these meetings, to provide information and to keep the discussion reasonably focused.

Psychiatric help

In some patients depression becomes severe and is not helped by ordinary counselling; occasionally there is the possibility of self-harm. In others there are abnormalities of behaviour that are not typical of the effects of head-injury and suggest an independent psychiatric condition. It is valuable to have the help of a psychiatrist who is familiar with head injury problems to help with the assessment and management of these patients.

Assessing progress

When a programme has been arranged for a patient, follow-up visits with the physician and neuropsychologist will be needed. Some of these will be informal, with a general discussion of symptoms and how the patient feels they are getting on. Others will be more structured and include follow-up neuropsychological testing; this is described in Chapter 8.

How patients themselves view their progress will change. In the early stages they sometimes lack insight and may deny the seriousness of their symptoms. Often this is followed by a quite sudden realistic appreciation of their problems; with this they may become depressed and their difficulties will seem greater than they are.

Keeping the patient informed about their progress is important, but this needs to be managed sensibly and factually. It is sometimes tempting to exaggerate improvement to make the patient feel better, but they could interpret this as license to cut short on their fatigue management, which would set them back instead of helping. If the patient has been an equal partner in the rehabilitation process they deserve to know the true situation, so that they can cooperate with their therapist and come up with a modification to the programme which will work better.

Whether the accident happened recently or months ago patients will want a prognosis, a time when they will be back to normal. In the authors' clinic we make sure that we talk about this at regular intervals in the support groups, pointing out how impossible it is to answer the question accurately. We emphasize that there are many factors involved in recovery apart from the sort of injury and the type of rehabilitation, and that all of them influence the amount of recovery that will occur and the time that it will take. We stress that they need to cope with how they are now, to take each day as it comes, and not to waste energy on focusing on some time in the future for which no one can give them a date.

Return to work

As progress is assessed, the stage will eventually be reached when return to work in some form can be considered. This will require a report from the rehabilitation workers that the patient has been involved with, a medical and neuropsychological review, and negotiations with an employer. It may be possible to consider return to the previous job, or another as a temporary measure may be more suitable.

The review will consider the following points.

(1) Is attention and concentration adequate? There is good correlation between work tolerance and appropriate neuropsychological tests, such as the PASAT (see Chapter 8).

(2) Under practical conditions can the patient hold their concentration for a sufficient time, and is fatigue adequately appreciated and managed? A sufficient estimate of this may be possible from the patient's description of what they have been doing on their own; a more satisfactory measure is a trial of work in a rehabilitation facility, if this can be arranged.

(3) Can the patient interact appropriately with other people in a work situation? Is irritability under good control? Again this may be judged from the account of the patient and their family, but observation at actual work may be needed when there is doubt.

(4) Are there significant problems with vision, balance, sense of smell, or sensitivity to noise?

The questions that will come up in negotiations with the prospective employer are the following.

(1) It will almost always be necessary to start with working part time. Is this acceptable, either with wages for time worked or unpaid as a work trial?

(2) Are there safety considerations? Are concentration and speed of reaction sufficient for safe and efficient work?

(3) Does the patient have to travel far to work and will the journeys to and from work add significantly to fatigue? Is the patient fit to drive to work?

(4) Can the patient's work be adequately supervised to begin with?

(5) Taking back an employee under these circumstances results in trouble and expense. Is there a way in which the community can recognize this?

If it is not possible to arrange for work with the old employer, another one may be able to meet the conditions. A trial at a less demanding job may be a more practical option.

When the patient's problems have been relatively mild these conditions will be fairly simple to meet. In other cases getting a patient placed in work may become a lengthy and frustrating process, and will place much stress on them, so that it is a time when they will need a great deal of support.

The patient who doesn't improve

Some patients show no progress, in spite of having a programme set up for them and being given help to run it. Difficulties crop up, appointments are not kept, and new symptoms may appear. Sometimes they have made progress and seem ready to start a work trial, then nothing that is arranged is suitable. If they do start work, before long it is found that they are not attending regularly or they say that the job is not suitable.

It is important to try at least once to sort out the reasons for this behaviour. The neuropsychological assessment should be checked; performance is likely to be impaired but may be inconsistent. The family and, if possible, someone independent should be asked about their performance before the accident. There may be a problem with personal relations which has been brought on by the accident. There may be some features of their behaviour which suggest a psychotic element, and if so a psychiatric opinion should be sought.

Unfortunately in many cases there will be no obvious cause except an inadequate personality. If counselling fails further rehabilitation is likely to be fruitless; one of the social agencies may be able to help them to change their lifestyle.

This picture is usually different from that of the deliberate malingerer, who is likely to complain consistently of a specific group of symptoms. The inconsistencies in the neuropsychological assessment are likely to be more clear cut; they are discussed further in Chapter 8. It should be remembered that sometimes this behaviour is a cry for help rather than a deliberate attempt to get compensation.

The needs of special groups

Some groups of patients, such as housewives, children, students, professional people, and executives, need special management. This is discussed in Chapter 11.

How is this organized?

If mild head injury is to be treated in a way that gets the patient back to normality and work as quickly as possible, and with the least expenditure on services and support, some degree of formal organization is necessary. Though hospital accident departments are only too aware of the number of patients with concussion that pass through their care, few have the facilities for following them up and many would not think it part of their function to do so. The small proportion of patients who do not recover swiftly or completely tend to be seen by general practitioners or neurologists who do not have a special interests or expertise in the problem and who lack ready access to the facilities for management; the problem is of course even greater in small communities. Obviously it is not possible to have a large number of specialist clinics, but in every area there should be a clear line of referral, well established with hospitals and general practitioners, first to a local person or group with an interest in the problem, and from them if needed to more sophisticated facilities elsewhere. This might be an established head injury centre, though their priorities tend to be the management of major injuries.

Though it should be possible in this way to arrange access to expert opinion for everyone who needs it, providing the daily treatment and support that is needed is more difficult. Travelling to a centre for help may be too tiring for it to be useful. A visiting team can set up a home programme, but frequent supervision is likely to be too expensive. Residential treatment, with weekends at home, may be ideal for some patients but again may be too expensive. There is no easy solution.

Staff – at the first contact

The function of the staff at the first contact is to make a diagnosis and to set up an initial treatment programme. A physician is needed with an understanding of the neurology of head injury and also of the primary and secondary behavioural changes which can accompany it. The assessment of the cognitive and behavioural symptoms falls to the neuro-psychologist. Theirs is the key role; assessing the cognitive changes of mild head injury and the secondary behavioural changes, detecting the subject who is not doing their best, and deciding on the most effective remedial measures require a high degree of expertise.

At the first contact diagnosis may involve other staff not primarily connected with the service. There will sometimes be need for an ophthalmologist, an otologist, a specialist in physical medicine, or a psychiatrist. It is helpful if there is one member of these disciplines who is prepared to take a special interest in these referrals.

Setting up the initial programme will require in addition the input of a social worker and occupational therapist and, perhaps, a speech therapist and a clinical psychologist.

Staff – later

When the first programme has been worked out and discussed with the patient, and if possible with their family as well, help will be needed to implement it. It is best if one person establishes a bond and provides the major input. Whatever their own training, they will need to borrow from the disciplines of occupational therapy, speech therapy, and clinical psychology as is appropriate and be able to refer problems to colleagues in other spheres if they are in difficulty. Later, when considering return to work, expertise with industrial placement will be needed.

Funding

Funding for management will depend on local circumstances, whether it is provided by an inclusive health system, partly or totally from insurance, or from what can be obtained by litigation. It is common experience that meeting the cost, from whatever source, takes constant effort and protection from discouragement.

This discouragement often takes the form of requests for proof that re-habilitation programmes are in fact of any help in reducing disability after MHI. This proof is very hard to find. Partly this is because of the difficulty in designing a suitably stringent experiment comparing a group that had received rehabilitation with one who had received none. Partly it is because of the ethical issues that are involved in withholding treatment if there is a likelihood that it could be of benefit. From the practical point of view it is because staff are under increasing pressure to deal with more and more cases for the same amount of funding, so that there are no spare resources of time and people to research what they are achieving. These issues are discussed by Cope (1995).

Other problems with assessment are illustrated in a recent study (Cicerone *et al.* 1996) where half a group of patients did and half did not show benefit from rehabilitation. Such a result is to be expected, given the individual variability in response to MHI, and the variability of the primary organic and secondary psychological consequences. Nevertheless it is worth continuing to try to establish the effectiveness of rehabilitation to a suitably scientific standard.

From the practical point of view we believe that the advantages of a programme of rehabilitation are convincingly demonstrated by the improvement of well-being of patients who have entered such a programme after living in limbo for months before they were directed to our clinic.

References and further reading

Cicerone, K. D., Smith, L. C., Ellmo, W., Mangel, H. R., Nelson, P., Chase, R. F., and Kalmar, K. (1996). Neuropsychological rehabilitation of mild traumatic brain injury. *Brain Injury,* **10**, 277–86.

Cope, D. N. (1995). The effectiveness of traumatic brain injury rehabilitation; a review. *Brain Injury,* **9**, 649–70.

Levin, H. S., Eisenberg, H. M., and Benton, A. L. (eds) (1989). *Mild head injury.* Oxford University Press, New York.

Rizzo, M. and Tranel, D. (eds) (1996) *Head injury and post concussive syndrome.* Churchill Livingstone, New York.
As mentioned in other chapters, this book provides a detailed account of many of the specialized areas of management of the PCS.

Robertson, I. H. (1994). Methodology in neuropsychological rehabilitation research (Editorial). *Neuropsychological Rehabilitation,* **4**, 1–6.

10
Medication

Introduction

The most pressing part of the management of MHI is to set up and support a practical daily programme which addresses cognitive and behavioural problems and the all-important factor of fatigue. Sometimes this is not enough and a patient's progress is halted by poor sleep, by irritability or impulsive behaviour, and particularly by depression. Early onset of fatigue may still be preventing the return to full-time work, and the patient may only be able to think constructively for the first few hours of the day.

In these situations it may be profitable to consider medication. Dealing with sleep, irritability, and depression can be relatively straightforward; fatigue and the enhancement of cognitive function are more difficult problems.

With so many neurochemical systems in the brain, interacting with each other in a complex way, it is only possible in a general way to relate clinical states to chemical function. Similarly there is available a multitude of drugs, each of which acts on one or more of the neurochemical systems with varying clinical responses. In treating head injury it is therefore wise to use a small range of drugs to deal with conditions that are well defined, and to know them well.

Sleep

In the early days after a head injury most patients will sleep deeply and for longer hours than usual. As they recover, often the pattern changes. They get to sleep, but wake after two or three hours, lie awake for a time, and then sleep uneasily until morning. Often this happens when the patient has recovered enough to have some insight and is concerned about the progress of their recovery. Support, reassurance, and so-called 'sleep hygiene' measures may be enough, but if sleep is still interrupted a short period of medication with a benzodiazepine such as temazepam should be tried. If this is not successful, amitriptyline 10–20 mg two hours before going to bed is likely to be effective. Before starting this, however, it should be considered whether the sleep problem is not a manifestation of depression, and whether this should not be the basis of treatment.

Depression

Many patients become depressed by the symptoms of MHI and the way they stop the normal enjoyment of life. If they had depressive tendencies before the accident the effect will be worse. Their depression may be obvious from what they say or how they behave, or it may show up in symptoms such as sleeplessness, failure to progress, or even a deterioration in performance (see Chapters 5, 8 and 9).

Medication will be needed if the symptoms do not resolve with counselling and support. The choice will be between a tricyclic antidepressant like amitriptyline or a serotonin reuptake inhibitor such as fluoxetine. Amitriptyline is more likely to be effective if one of the types of headache is present, or if sleep is a problem. Its disadvantages are the anticholinergic effects of a dry mouth and visual blurring, daytime sedation, and the impairment of cognitive function, which is more marked when it is used in head injury patients than in other depressed people. Many people dislike it to begin with but get used to it; if it is to have the best chance of being acceptable the dose should be minimal at first – 10–25 mg at night, and then increased only slowly; head injury patients will often complain of impaired function when the dose exceeds 50 mg.

Fluoxetine has the advantage of minimal anticholinergic effects and much less impairment of cognitive function. It is not so effective when pain or sleep disturbance is a factor, and may cause nausea or agitation.

Many of the other antidepressants with more or less similar profiles are suitable; which is chosen will depend on local factors and the personal experience of the prescriber.

Impulsive and aggressive behaviour

This is not common after mild head injury but it does occur. If it is a significant handicap and does not respond to counselling or a behaviour modification programme the first choice is an anticonvulsant, specifically carbamazepine or valproate. The dose needed will usually be considerably less than that needed to control seizures.

Fatigue and cognitive function

Fatigue, poor concentration, and slow thinking will be managed to begin with by arranging limited periods of activity and learning to forestall the onset of fatigue with obligatory periods of rest. With this programme most people will regain useful function in time. Some stop improving, perhaps when they are doing part of their normal work but not the full load. In these people it may be worth trying medication to improve cognitive function and extend the time for which it is possible to work. There are two pharmacological approaches, to increase arousal and to support the cholinergic neural activity that is important in memory and information processing.

The medication most often used to increase arousal is methylphenidate (Ritalin), familiar to most from its use in children with attention deficit. As these patients often function reasonably for the first two or three hours a day it may be helpful to give the first dose mid-morning and another in the afternoon; administration later in the day may interfere with sleep. The gain and the side-effects vary from patient to patient, and the dose needs a good deal of adjustment to the needs of the individual. Some patients will find the medication worth while, a typical response being the ability to extend what was a half day's work to an hour or two in the afternoon. Unfortunately many patients find little benefit or are put off by the side-effects.

Medication intended to increase the availability of acetylcholine has become an important goal in the treatment of the Alzheimer group of dementias and could be of help to patients with a long term stationary cognitive impairment. Cholinesterase inhibitors such as Donepezil or Rivastigmine may prove to be of value, but so far there have been no useful trials on MHI patients. Compounds affecting other neurochemical systems have been tried but none seem to be sufficiently well explored to be adopted for clinical use.

11
Special cases

Introduction

In a previous chapter we described the general principles of management of the later effects of mild head injury. Some groups of patients have special needs, and it is essential to understand what these are if the patients are to be properly cared for.

Children

Children have special problems with mild head injury. Younger children may not lose consciousness at the time of the injury but may go into a drowsy state later. Rarely they may suffer temporary cortical blindness. In the first few weeks older children may experience symptoms like those seen in adults, with disturbed behaviour and difficulty with school work. In both instances there is the possibility that mild injury can result in long term cognitive and behavioural problems.

Children up to six

Mild head injury is common in children in this age group, usually as the result of a fall. There may be a definite loss of consciousness, but often they only appear stunned and then after a moment or two will begin to talk or cry. In the next few minutes or up to an hour or so they may be subdued or irritable. Sometimes then, often after vomiting, they will drift into what seems to be a deep sleep. In this state they will react to stimuli but cannot be properly wakened. After an hour or more they will become responsive again, though they are usually fretful and not themselves for a time. Often there will be concern that there may be an intracranial bleed; however, the child can be roused to some extent, the pupil reactions are normal and there are no other neurological or pulse and blood pressure changes. If in doubt a CT scan will be done and will be normal.

A rarer event, which can occur in both this age group and in older children, is the onset after an interval of up to an hour or so of cortical blindness. The child will quite suddenly say that everything has gone dark and that they cannot see. Pupil reactions are normal and there are no other neurological abnormalities. The blindness remains for up to an hour or two, and then clears with no lasting impairment. The possible causes of these two syndromes are discussed in Chapter 3.

When they have recovered from the acute effects of injury most young children will be weepy and irritable for a few days but then over a week or two will return to their normal behaviour. A few will stay like this for longer, perhaps several weeks, and occasionally there can be a lasting change in behaviour.

When changes persist after a mild injury it may be difficult to be sure what is the cause. At this age there is a rapid development of social and cognitive skills which may be disturbed by a number of factors, of which the accident may be only one. Neuropsychological assessment, which could be diagnostic in older children, is difficult at this age. Because of this there has been reluctance to accept that mild injuries can have a direct effect on cognitive performance in younger children. However, recent work on the development of some visual skills after mild injury have shown that though there may be no detectable evidence of impairment immediately, the orderly sequence of development may have been disturbed (Wrightson *et al.* 1995). A year or more later definite changes may be detected that can affect abilities such as those of learning to read or of learning mathematics. One well controlled longitudinal study showed that when mildly head injured children were given a test of mathematical ability at the age of ten years, those in whom the accident occurred when they were aged five or six years performed less well than those injured when they were older (Bijur *et al.* 1990).

If the injury has been anything more than minimal the chance of late effects should be discussed with the parents. This is a sensitive area and they should be seen by an experienced member of staff. It should be explained that sometimes, skills such as reading can be slower to develop, but that with proper help this can be corrected. As far as they can, parents should keep a check on how their child is progressing, and should ask the kindergarten or primary school teacher to look at the child's pre-reading and reading performance so that they can have extra help early on if it is needed.

Children aged seven and upwards

Injuries in this age group are less likely to be due to falls; road traffic accidents and, in older children, sports are the most common causes. In the acute stage the pattern of symptoms is more like that in adults, and management is similar. Later there can be special problems with getting back to school and making progress there.

Often children in this age group, like adults, will go through a period of a few days to several weeks in which they are not themselves. To begin with they are often lethargic and irritable. When they seem fit to return to school they may find it difficult to cope with the demands of work and play. In most cases they settle back to normal in a week or two, but if they are slow to recover teachers may not understand what has happened and label them as 'not trying'. Though they do in time recover, the label may stick and become a self-fulfilling prophecy.

Again in this age group it has not yet been thoroughly established that long term cognitive impairment can occur. Evidence for this is difficult to obtain because there are so many other potent factors which affect personality and school achievement. There is, however, no reason to suppose that if mild injury can cause structural lesions and cognitive impairment in adults, children should be immune. If there is a difference in outcome it would need to be due to children having an efficient mechanism for compensation, and indeed some theorists maintain that this is the case. However, as in the younger children, the acquisition of adult skills depends on the orderly sequence of developmental steps and it may be that impairment, even for a short period, may interfere with one of these steps and so have long term consequences.

Management

In the acute stage it is important to be aware of the common delayed effect seen in younger children, and of the rare complications such as cortical blindness.

It is important that parents are told that it is normal for their child to be easily tired, irritable, and perhaps tearful over the next few days after an injury, and that this stage should be over before they are sent back to school. Even then, though the child may seem to be behaving reasonably normally, it is likely that they will still be having some difficulty with concentration and attention, and teachers should be aware of this. In most cases they will have settled back to normal after a week or two.

In some cases the child may take longer to recover. Though they seem fit enough to go back to school, when they get there they cannot fit in with the programme. They may be easily distractable, so that there is a problem with behaviour. A picture often seen is that they manage reasonably well with the early periods in the day, but then lose concentration and cannot cope with the work. It may be sufficient for a period of a week or two to limit the hours at school, perhaps with the child attending until midday or even only to the mid-morning break, and then slowly increasing the period at school as performance improves. The children are often easily distractable, and this may lead to disruptive behaviour in the class.

When problems continue for more than a week or two it is important to deal with them effectively to avoid secondary changes. A neuropsychological assessment is desirable as a guide to further management, and special help with teaching should be arranged.

In some schools the problems that occur with head injury have not been well understood or managed. Children who did not return to normal performance quickly have been regarded as slacking, and either pushed harder or disciplined. Again some boys' schools have made light of concussion sustained in sport and coaches have insisted on a return to play within days of the injury. In the authors' region the school nurses were concerned about this lack of understanding, and asked for a statement that could be used in their schools to increase staff awareness. Readers may find the result, printed in Appendix 3, useful in their area.

Talking to parents about the possibility of long term effects is a sensitive issue and may result in unnecessary anxiety. Any discussion of this sort should be with an experienced member of staff. It is sensible to mention possible problems in the case of pre-school children, so that reading problems can be anticipated, and parents of older children should make sure that problems are being dealt with properly at school.

High school and university students

Young people in senior school and university probably depend on cognitive competence more than any other group, so that its impairment while they are recovering from the effects of a mild head injury may have a catastrophic effect, particularly if it occurs at a critical time in the academic year such as the run up to an examination. They are often reluctant to admit to their deficiencies to begin with and often fail to take advice about sensible management. When their problems can no longer be ignored there may be a swing to depression and destructive decisions such as abandoning their studies. As well a the ordinary management, a counsellor is needed who is familiar with academic requirements, together with a good liaison with school and university authorities. It may be possible to reduce the load by postponing some courses, and if exams are imminent, they may be able to sit them if extra time is allowed, or aegrotat passes may be applied for.

Executives and professional people

Similar problems arise with executives and professional people. They need to make decisions based on multiple factors, to switch from problem to problem, to follow conversation round a group, and to work long hours under stress, classical areas of difficulty after a mild head injury. Often they go back to work too soon, either not having had good advice about the problems they may meet, or ignoring it. They then find they cannot cope, and neither they nor the people they work with understand what has happened. Destructive situations develop rapidly. Such patients are often hard to counsel, resist advice, and do not fit in with the usual support sessions. The counsellor should try to persuade them to follow the same course as other people, to start with a period of complete rest and then return to work, part time at first, only when neuropsychological test results are satisfactory. There is, however, a problem here, inherent in assessing high functioning people, that a score that is in the normal range for the whole population is significantly below normal for them (see Chapter 8). They should be impressed with the importance of managing fatigue and a formal daily programme should be followed. It will be a help to rearrange their working day, scheduling the tough decisions for the first couple of hours in the morning. They should be encouraged to delegate as much as possible to a personal assistant. Even then the situation is likely to be fragile, and is at the mercy of a business crisis, a late night, or a family argument, which can set them back for weeks. They are particularly vulnerable to the 'I can do it if I try harder' danger.

Patients in this and the previous group will often be helped by the booklet 'Getting back to work at the desk', included in Appendix 5.

Older people

Recovery from the effects of mild head injury is slower and usually less complete in older people, with the effect being seen to some degree even in people in their 40s. Again those whose work depends on cognitive function are likely to be affected to a greater extent. Fatigue is even more of a problem than in younger people. If they lose their job because of the injury the chance of getting another one at their age may seem slim. Depression may become an important factor. In the older patient, in their 60s or late 50s the best advice for the counsellor to give them may be to accept a long term disability and to consider a partial or complete retirement. It may make the situation more acceptable if it is emphasized that experience, judgement, and wisdom are intact and that it is only the demand for speed and endurance which cannot be met.

Long term reduction of capacity

This is a familiar problem after severe head injury, but it can also follow minor injury, and some patients remain for long periods with a disability sufficient to prevent them playing their full part in life. They may have been under observation from the time of their injury, or have presented after a period in which the origin of their symptoms has been uncertain.

There may be deficits which make specific cognitive rehabilitation useful, but the important strategies for coping with everyday life are those of careful organization of the daily programme, fatigue management, and supportive counselling. Provided an acceptable programme can be worked out, the patient may be able to live a reasonably productive life.

Post-traumatic stress disorder

Post-traumatic stress disorder (PTSD) is now recognized as a disabling condition that can occur as a reaction to horrifying or life-threatening situations such as war zones, natural disasters, or extraordinary violence. The characteristics are intrusive 'flashbacks' of the incident, recurrent nightmares, and avoidance of thoughts and situations that are related to it. The state of high anxiety that is produced leads to cognitive changes and mood disorders, including sleep problems, fatigue, irritability, problems in concentrating, and amnesia for the event itself. Most of these are indistinguishable from the symptoms that follow MHI, and it is not surprising that there was a move some years ago to explain all MHI and PCS complaints as PTSD. Such an extreme view is no longer tenable.

However, there can be no argument that motor vehicle accidents, assaults, or falls can all be classified as traumatic and life-threatening situations. It would therefore be predicted that PTSD would develop in a proportion of cases in which they had caused a head injury, especially if the diagnosis was made on the basis of the symptoms they described. The incidence of traumatic brain injury cases which are classified as having PTSD varies markedly, depending on the theoretical bias of the investigator. Thus where PTA, information processing deficits, fatigue, and poor concentration are labelled as PTSD, the proportion is high. Where these symptoms are not taken to have a differential diagnostic value, the proportion is very low, usually around 2–5 per cent.

One of the criteria for PTSD is that the condition has persisted for at least a month after the traumatic event. However, an additional diagnostic category has now been included in the DSM-IV to cover the period from two days to a month. According to Bryant and Harvey (Bryant 1996, Bryant and Harvey 1996), acute stress disorder (ASD) is characterized by exposure to serious trauma followed by dissociation, re-experiencing the trauma, avoidance, and anxiety. These authors examined a group of patients injured in motor vehicle accidents early after their admission to hospital. In the patients who had not had a head injury they found that 13 per cent met the criteria for ASD. Two of the dissociative symptoms, amnesia for the event and slow reaction times, are typical after-effects of head injury and were not used in evaluating the 92 head-injured admissions who all had durations of PTA of less than 24 h. Even so, 5 per cent of this group met the criteria for ASD.

In contrast, the argument has been put forward by Sbordone (Sbordone and Liter 1995) amongst others that PTSD cannot occur in cases of traumatic brain injury (TBI), because these patients are amnesic for the accident and thus have no frightening or life-threatening event to recall. However, there is an increasing body of evidence that PTSD is found even after severe TBI, possibly because of 'islands' of memory during the amnesic period, and possibly because of 'pseudomemories', which have been shown to be as compelling as actual memories of an event (Bryant 1996, Bryant and Harvey 1996).

It is reasonable to suppose therefore that mildly head injured patients with a minimal duration of PTA would also be likely to develop the stress reaction, and this has been shown to be the case in several studies, with an incidence again of around 2–5 per cent, depending on the diagnostic criteria used. This has led to the suggestion that when PCS is prolonged it may be more accurately diagnosed as PTSD. Given that most workers consider that PCS results from a combination of 'organic' factors arising from damage to the CNS and secondary 'psychogenic' factors which develop in reaction to the primary injury, this may indeed be the case.

There are, however, some reports which question whether post-traumatic stress symptoms occurring after MHI might better be regarded as a subgroup of PTSD, since vivid re-experiences and flashbacks are much less frequent than in other PTSD populations. Similarly, Ohry *et al.* (1996) note that combat stress reaction casualties have higher levels of intrusive than avoidance symptoms, while their head-injured cases showed the opposite ratio.

Apart from the difficulties with symptom overlap there are other problems of unravelling the issue, including the contribution of neurological symptoms such as vertigo and diplopia, which make it difficult for the patients not to be continually reminded of the accident, and so not to be able to put it behind them and get on with their life.

For practical purposes, however, this controversy is a non-issue. While the difference between the aetiologies of PTSD and PCS is of academic interest, and though it is argued by some that the issue is important in planning effective treatment, we believe that for a patient referred for rehabilitation after MHI the question is irrelevant. The aim of their rehabilitation is education and reassurance, management of stress, of fatigue, and of anger, and frequent monitoring of progress (see Chapter 9). We consider that the priority is to establish the presence and extent of MHI symptoms and to try to prevent secondary stress developing. This is very similar to programmes designed for PTSD, for instance that described by McGrath (1997) for a patient with PTSD after MHI. For a fuller discussion of specific treatment for PTSD the article by Miller (1993) can be consulted.

There have been some positive results from the examination of the relationship between the two conditions. Of practical importance is the examination of factors that are associated with the development of ASD and PTSD. These include a past history of psychiatric disorder, previous traumas, life stress, and gender – the PTSD group contains a higher proportion of females than would be expected from their distribution in the total number of head injuries. These are factors which also tend to be important in the development of a persistent PCS.

The distinction between the PCS and PTSD can be of medicolegal importance. When symptoms which resemble PTSD form a significant part of the disability, insurance companies may claim that circumstances preceding the accident are wholly or partly responsible and that therefore their liability is diminished. It may be easier for them to make this case with the PTSD than with the PCS. We do not believe that this is a valid reason for withholding compensation. As we describe in Chapter 13, the essence of the claimant's rebuttal will be that they were functioning well before the accident, and that whatever changes have occurred must be ascribed to it.

A full discussion of the more atypical responses to head trauma, such as hysterical reactions or psychosomatic or dissociative disorders, is beyond the scope of this book. However, these issues are covered by Lezac (1996), which has a useful background section, and Ponsford *et al.* (1995), which examines the effect of such disorders on attempts to apply remedial behaviour therapy to head-injured patients.

References and further reading

Bijur, P.A., Haslum, M., and Golding, J. (1990). Cognitive and behavioural sequelae of mild head injury in children. *Paediatrics*, **86**, 337–44.
This study concludes that mild head injury does not in general affect the cognitive status of children at age 10, but did find that injury at ages 5–7 significantly impaired proficiency in mathematics.

Bryant, R. A. (1996). Traumatic memories and pseudomemories following traumatic brain injury. In *International perspectives in traumatic brain injury*, (ed. Ponsford, *et al.*). Australian Academic Press.

Bryant, R. A. and Harvey, A. G. (1996). Acute stress disorder following traumatic brain injury. In *International perspectives in traumatic brain injury*, (ed. Ponsford, J., Snow, P., and Anderson, V.). Australian Academic Press, Melbourne.

Lezac, M. D. (1996). *Neuropsychological assessment*, (3rd edn). Oxford University Press, New York.

McGrath, J. (1997). Cognitive impairment associated with post-traumatic stress disorder and minor head injury: a case report. *Neuropsychological Rehabilitation*, **7**, 231–9.

Miller, L. (1993). The 'trauma' of head trauma: clinical, neuropsychological and forensic aspects of post-traumatic stress syndromes in brain injury. *Journal of Cognitive Rehabilitation*, **July/August**, 18–29.

Ohry, A., Rattok, J., and Solomon, Z. (1996). Post-traumatic stress disorder in brain-injury patients. *Brain Injury*, **10**, 687–95.

Ponsford, J., Sloan, S., and Snow, P. (1995). *Traumatic brain injury: rehabilitation for everyday adaptive living*. Lawrence Erlbaum Associates, Hove.

Sbordone, R. J. and Liter, J. C. (1995). Mild traumatic brain injury does not produce post-traumatic stress disorder. *Brain Injury,* **9**, 405–12.

Snoek, J. W., Minderhoud, J. M., and Wilmink, J. T. (1984). Delayed deterioration following mild head injury in children. *Brain,* **107**, 15–36.

This describes several forms of deterioration including cortical blindness.

Wrightson, P., McGinn, V., and Gronwall, D. (1995). Mild head injury in preschool children: evidence that it can be associated with a persisting cognitive defect. *Journal of Neurology, Neurosurgery and Psychiatry,* **59**, 375–80.

This suggests that minimal concussion in young children can affect the orderly development of skills and lead to later cognitive defects.

12
Sports injuries

Introduction

In the authors' city sport is responsible for about 20 per cent of the head injuries seen at emergency departments and allowed home, and for about 7 per cent of those admitted to hospital. Sports injuries themselves are usually mild but several considerations give them a special importance. The player will want to continue playing, at once or later, and so will risk another injury. Further injury within a week or two of the first risks a catastrophic reaction. Multiple minor injuries can cause a permanent loss of brain function.

Sports people have a strong drive to succeed and have themselves usually accepted the possibility of injury. They do not want to be seen to give in, especially to an injury such as concussion, for which there is no external evidence. In professional sport, players and managers lose money when someone is unable to play. At every stage there is therefore a strong motive to minimize concern over mild head injury. The more reputable governing bodies have set down clear rules to cover the response to head injury, but at the local level there is often resistance to applying them.

The issues at stake are whether the player is well enough to go on playing immediately after an injury to the head, how soon they should be allowed to play again if they have been laid off, and whether after more than one or two head injuries they should stop playing.

The greatest number of injuries occurs in one of the football codes, and the next section deals with these. An account of the considerations in other sports follows.

Football injuries

Diagnosis of concussion on the football field

The first person to assess the injured person is the referee. They may be supported later by a doctor, but the prime responsibility is theirs. The referee has no problem in making a diagnosis if the player has lost consciousness and he sees them in this state; the player must be removed from the field and treated in the same way as for a head injury in any other situation. There should be no question of their resuming play.

Often the situation is not so clear. There has been an injury which has made the player lose touch with the game, but it may not be plain to other players or the referee that there has been a loss of consciousness. They see the player lying on the ground or trying to stand, confused and ataxic. If this condition continues for more than a minute or so, there is again no doubt that they must leave the game. There is a problem, however, if the player seems to return to normal more quickly and says that they are ready to resume play.

When there is doubt whether the player should continue, the referee should have available a simple and unequivocal protocol that he can use to make an administrative decision, which does not depend on special medical or first aid experience. The protocol can be printed as part of the referee's equipment on the field. A form which has been found practical is the following.

Concussion: Notes for referees

There has been concussion if
- the player is seen to have been unconscious for even the shortest time;
- the player was unresponsive for even the shortest time (i.e. did not open eyes, speak, or get up at once);
- the player was confused for even the shortest time – didn't know what to do, which way to play, where he was;
- the player was unsteady on his feet, reeling, or unable to hold the ball;
- the player showed spasms or convulsions.

The player must be able
- to tell you
  the day of the week, the month, the year;
  the name of the other team;
  the score and if it is first or second half;
- to walk steadily heel-to-toe.

Concussion often destroys judgement.
Do not allow a player to influence you: his health and the reputation of the game are at stake.

This protocol does not make use of memory tests. These are important in the full assessment of mild head injury, but not practical here. Retrograde amnesia may not develop for a few minutes after the injury, and testing for post-traumatic amnesia takes five minutes at the least (see Chapter 3), so neither is suitable for on-the-field use.

There will be some variation in the way these rules are applied, depending on whether a major match is being played by professionals or it is a local match or a school game. It is probably safe for fit adult players to return to the game if they pass the referee's tests. Players under 16, or the less fit (such as older players in a friendly game), should probably not play on after a head injury that halts the game, even if they pass the tests.

The risks of playing on

If players are allowed to continue without careful screening, a proportion will still be mildly confused and ataxic. The reflexes which normally protect against injury will be less effective. Players are likely to be less expert and of less use, or even a handicap, to their team. A second head injury is possible, with a small risk of the second injury syndrome, described below.

Other opinions and other codes

The literature on injuries in various football codes describes different definitions and various degrees of head injury. The precautions described above have been, for a number of years, reasonably well accepted by the Rugby Union code in the authors' country. The risk of injury is different in other codes, probably being least in Association football and greatest in some of the USA codes. Especially in the USA, more complex classifications of the immediate state are current. One that has been widely used is that proposed by the Colorado Medical Society. This defines three grades of concussion. In grade 1 there is confusion but no loss of consciousness and no amnesia. The player is sidelined and observed for 20 minutes and if there is no deterioration and no amnesia develops they are allowed to return to the game. In grade 2 there is confusion with amnesia but again no loss of consciousness. These players do not return to the game, but are observed for a period to detect any developing signs. In grade 3 concussion there has been loss of consciousness, and it is recommended that the player be transferred to hospital for observation. It is, however, questionable whether the distinction between grades 1 and 2 is valid, considering the difficulty in estimating amnesia when this is of short duration, and the system may be sensitive to commercial pressures. It is likely that a simple system is safest for the player, and this should be the major consideration. (A description of some of the major schemes of assessment is given in *Football injuries of the head and neck*; National Health and Medical Research Council 1994.)

Ready to play again? – Short term considerations

There are two separate issues, which should not be confused. The first and dominant issue is the risk of a catastrophic second injury. A player who has had a head injury up to three weeks or so previously, though usually not more than ten days, receives a second mild injury, and within an hour becomes deeply unconscious. Investigations show a tensely swollen brain, usually with some subdural bleeding. In most cases the signs of cerebral compression progress to brain death within 36 h. The mechanism is uncertain, but is likely to involve a vascular reaction. In some of the cases reported the player has been unwell at the time of the second injury, either with a headache or general malaise, and it is likely that some viral illnesses predispose to the syndrome (see Chapter 3).

There are two practical problems. The first is that there is insufficient information on the magnitude of the risk. The number of cases described in the literature is small, but many neurosurgeons are aware of instances which have not been reported. Probably all that can be said is that the consequences can be so serious that the possibility must be taken into account.

The second problem is deciding when it is safe to play again. The reported cases have almost all occurred within three weeks of the first injury, and mostly within a fortnight, so that laying off a player for this period is an adequate safeguard. Where a player wants to return before the three weeks are up there is no certain way of telling whether it is safe. Most of the cases of second injury deterioration have had some symptoms before the event, and so anyone with headache or other post-concussion symptoms should certainly not play. A recent viral illness may increase the risk and is another contraindication. Brain imaging may not be helpful, and the authors know of two cases where a CT scan was normal before the deterioration. If it is important to resume play, a genuine absence of symptoms, a normal neuropsychological assessment, and possibly a normal MR scan would make it reasonably safe.

A further issue is the effectiveness of the player. The ability to make rapid decisions is the essence of most sports; the most solidly documented effect of mild head injury is slowing of this ability. This means that there is an increased risk of another accident, which in some sports such as motor racing or hang gliding could be fatal. However, after most mild injuries speed has recovered by three weeks, though in a minority, not characterized by any particular feature of the injury, the slowing will persist as part of a post-concussion syndrome.

A practical policy, which has been adopted in a number of sports, is to forbid participation for three weeks after a mild head injury. This is a reasonable safeguard against second injury deterioration and allows most players to recover their ability to make rapid decisions. At the end of the period it is sensible to require a medical examination before resuming play. This will identify those who still have physical symptoms such as headache or impaired balance and coordination, who should certainly not resume play until they are clear. It may not, however, detect those who are still slow but otherwise well, who may be at risk. It would not be practical to make a formal neuropsychological assessment of everyone before they resume playing, but it may be sensible before important matches or in other sports such as motor racing or hang gliding where speed of reaction is critical or failure particularly dangerous. As a practical compromise, assessment of choice reaction times could be done in the doctor's office. This will give some objective information on fitness to resume the sport. More is said about this in Chapter 8.

Considering the large number of players who suffer mild head injuries, and the considerable number who play again early against advice, the incidence of serious problems is small. However, when they do occur they are so dramatic and damaging to the individual and to the sport that its prevention is thought to be worth a great deal of inconvenience.

Returning to play – long term consideration

Most sports people would take it that a single mild head injury would have no lasting effect, but we know that this is not entirely true. In Chapter 5 we described how a proportion of fit young people who had returned to work soon after their injury were still aware of a fall-off in performance three months later, and how a small number still felt an effect after two years. Ordinary tests of cognitive function might not show any abnormalities, but under conditions of stress such as mild hypoxia they could perform less well.

There is also good evidence that a further injury will add to an existing deficit, and if there are several more the effect may become obvious, with slowing of reactions, difficulty in making decisions, and lack of insight. Surveys of sports people have shown that many of them have seen this happening and want to limit their risks. Others choose not to act in their own best interests or are subject to other pressures, and go on playing in spite of repeated injury.

To protect players from themselves and from external pressures, governing bodies of sports need to have a formal code which recognizes these dangers. A reasonable protocol is that a player may return to the game at the recommended time after the first head injury, but if there is a further injury they should not play again that season. An injury in the following season is taken as a warning, and if there is a further injury that season it is a strong indication to stop contact sports.

As with the stand down after a single injury a player may question the advice to give up contact sports. Can neuropsychological tests say reliably that function is either preserved or seriously at risk? Certainly in a proportion of players in this situation, tests on a single occasion will show a definite impairment that would support advice to give up play. Others will perform within normal limits, but these are wide; a player who started with superior abilities may have deteriorated, but still be within the normal range. Serial assessments such as have been carried out in some research projects may be the only way to be certain, but are not practical for general use. An MR scan may sometimes show structural abnormalities, though our knowledge of their significance is still imperfect.

If the regulations of the particular games code do not specify a mandatory prohibition of further play after so many injuries, the only course is to make all the facts known to the players, together with the best advice, and to leave them to make the decision. Unfortunately a minority of players will continue in spite of this warning.

Younger players

Head injuries do occur in school football, though less often than in adult play, and the same general rules about restriction of play apply. There are, however, two areas of concern. The first is that the effect of the injury on the ability to learn may be more serious than that on the established capacities in older people, so that greater care is needed. The second is that in some schools there is either a macho attitude to injury or ignorance of the possible effects of head injury on performance, and sometimes both.

It is important therefore that people concerned with sports medicine exert what influence they can on teaching staff and school or public health nurses, so that the rules of return to play which hold for adult codes are observed in schools, and that teachers make sure that pupils who have had a head injury are watched for any adverse effects that may make their learning difficult. An information sheet which has been used to help and inform school authorities is included in Appendix 3.

Boxing

In boxing matches, head punches play an important part in winning, as they affect the opponent's performance more surely than body blows. The local impact force of punches over the cranial vault is reduced by the gloves and by a helmet, if it is worn, but impacts of this sort are less likely to cause structural damage. The effect is much greater when the punches result in rotational acceleration of the head, for example when they land on the side of the jaw, and it is this that can finish a fight, either by the stupefaction produced by a cumulation of minor injuries or a knockout.

If blows to the head of this sort can produce temporary neurological dysfunction that is obvious to the onlooker, is there evidence that they cause lasting damage? There is no doubt that many professional boxers have been damaged, resulting in a form of dementia, 'dementia pugilistica', and a parkinsonian syndrome, or both. In the earlier years of the century professionals fought up to 200 contests, and around a half eventually showed signs of one of these syndromes, in many cases as they aged and years after they had stopped boxing. Recently few have taken part in more than 50 major contests, but there is still a high incidence of neurological abnormality, which appears to depend primarily on the number of bouts, with knockouts not being essential in producing the damage.

Do amateur boxers run the same risks? Amateur boxing has become closely controlled. Medical examination before the fight is mandatory (though what it purports to detect other than acute illnesses is not apparent). Helmets are worn. The number of rounds is limited to three, referees are instructed to stop the fight if it seems that there is neurological impairment, and there is a compulsory stand-down period after a fight has been stopped for this reason. In spite of this it is said that around 5 per cent of fights still end with a knockout.

It is still uncertain whether, in amateurs, these precautions are effective in preventing subtle but significant neurological damage. The doubt has generated a number of investigations. Neurological examination has sometimes shown abnormalities in balance and coordination, but not consistently. Laboratory tests – EEGs, evoked potentials, and CT scans – have generally not been helpful, though in one study SPECT scans showed abnormalities of blood flow in the basal ganglia. At the time of writing MR scans had not been done sufficiently often to contribute. A particular concern is that even amateur boxing when young may predispose to an Alzheimer type of dementia in later life, especially in those genetically predisposed by the possession of the ApoE e4 allele.

Neuropsychological testing has been generally accepted as being most likely to show up any damage that might be present, using the tests that have been shown to be sensitive to other forms of mild injury. Here again the findings have not yet been definitive, though there is a strong tendency for boxers to perform less well in the more sensitive tests, with deficiencies being greater in those who had fought more contests.

The balanced view would seem to be that there is a continuum of damage from the gross changes seen in professional boxers to minimal abnormalities in amateurs who have recently begun to box. Those who support boxing believe that this minimal damage is not significant in the boxer's future. Others see the risk of any avoidable loss of cognitive capacity as indefensible, particularly as minor loss in young boxers may become more important as they grow older.

There is particular concern about boxing in young people. In a large survey of American boxing, 43 per cent of the amateur boxers examined were aged 13–15, with 15 per cent of them having started boxing at the age of 10 or less; 28 per cent were at least one grade behind in school. It is impossible on the data available to say whether scholastically impaired children chose boxing to compensate for their failures or if boxing made them fail. There is, however, no doubt that even mild injuries may impair the ability to learn.

The American Medical Association and the British Medical Association have said that boxing should be abolished, for both practical and ethical reasons. Some countries have outlawed it. It continues, however, in both professional and amateur forms, to be highly popular in many countries. Those interested in sports injuries need to make their views known.

Horse riding

Mild head injury is not uncommon in people who ride for pleasure. Helmets are usually worn; these give protection from impact injuries in falls, but as in the case of boxing are less effective in reducing the effect of angular acceleration.

Concussion is common in both professional and amateur jockeys. As in other sports there is strong pressure to minimize the consequences. The rules for stand-down and multiple injuries should be similar to those for footballers and these are laid down by many racing authorities.

Golf

Injuries from the swinging club and the driven ball are surprisingly common (in Glasgow said to be the commonest sports injury needing neurosurgical attention). Apart from the occasional depressed fracture from a clubhead, they are due to high velocity impacts on the scalp, which can cause local cerebral contusions and subdural bleeding. It is important to realize that these can occur without loss of consciousness, but with a persisting neuropsychological disability due to local cortical damage.

Other sports

Almost all sports carry a risk of physical injury, and in many head injuries are common, often associated with damage to the cervical spine; gymnasts may be particularly liable to this form of injury. A small proportion of patients will have persistent problems and will need the management described earlier. However, only a few sports, such as football and boxing, carry a significant risk of repeated injury.

Further reading

Butler, R. J., Forsythe, W. I., Beverly, D. W., and Adams, L. M. (1993). A prospective controlled investigation of the cognitive effects of amateur boxing. *Journal of Neurology, Neurosurgery and Psychiatry,* **56**, 1055–61.

A well designed study which reports definite effects on cognitive function in the early days after fights, but with marked improvement on retest later. The impairment correlated with the number of blows to the head. It is surprising that the authors do not appear to be concerned about the long term effects.

Kelly, J. P., Nichols, J. S., Filley, C. M., Lillehei, K. O., Rubinstein, D., and Kleinschmidt-DeMasters, B. K. (1991). Concussion in sports: guidelines for the prevention of catastrophic outcome. *Journal of the American Medical Association*, **266**, 2867–9.

This reports cases of catastrophic second injury and discusses the rules needed to minimize the risk. it lists many useful references.

Kemp, P. M., Houston, A. S., Macleod, M. A., and Pethybridge, R. J. (1995). Cerebral perfusion and psychometric testing in military amateur boxers and controls. *Journal of Neurology, Neurosurgery and Psychiatry*, **59**, 368–74.

SPECT studies showed persisting abnormalities after boxing, with some correlation with neuropsychological testing.

National health and Medical Research Council (1994). *Football injuries of the head and neck*. Australian Government Publishing Service, Canberra.

Though this may not be easily available, it contains valuable comparisons of the codes of various sports as they cover return to play and then the prevention of further injury.

Stewart, W. F., Gordon, B., Selnes, O., Bandeen-Roche, K., Zeger, S., Tusa, R. J. *et al.* (1994). Prospective study of central nervous system function in amateur boxers in the United States. *American Journal of Epidemiology*, **139**, 573–88.

A large scale study, notable for the young age of many of the boxers and their lowered academic performance.

Wrightson, P. and Gronwall, D. (1980). Attitudes to concussion in young New Zealand men. *New Zealand Medical Journal*, **92**, 359–61.

13
Legal aspects

Introduction

An important responsibility of the team managing a patient with head injury is to make sure as soon as possible what funds will be available to cover the costs of treatment and loss of earnings. Unfortunately the amount and quality of rehabilitation that is available may depend on this. Therefore when it becomes evident that there is no or insufficient cover by private insurance or other sources, the patient and family will need to seek legal advice, the issue being whether there has been fault and whether it is likely that it will be possible to recover damages. The sooner this is done the better, both to obtain funding for treatment and because the investigation of the circumstances of the accident will be easier.

In the cases of mild head injury the situation is rather different. At first most patients will be expected to recover completely in a short time, and it may be several months before it is realized that there are serious problems and that funds will be needed for prolonged rehabilitation and income support.

The medical input at this stage will be to advise the chosen lawyer on the possible degree of disability and how long it is likely to be before this can be properly assessed. This may be difficult; severe injuries tend to follow a pattern, but in mild cases there is so much variation in the rate of progress and the outcome that predictions may be no more than a guess. The most that can be done may be to estimate a minimum further period of disability and to review the situation at the end of this. The doctor will, however, be able to certify that the patient is at the time unable to function normally because of the injury and to give a reasonable minimum further period of disability, and this may make it possible to commence an action and perhaps to secure some interim payment.

Obtaining legal advice

It is essential to consult a solicitor or attorney who is experienced in brain injury litigation, and if possible one who has a special interest in mild head injuries. Just as these demand specialized medical care, so do they need specialized legal representation. What will be obtained on the patient's behalf will have a long-term impact on some aspects of the quality of their life, and the more experienced the lawyer is the better the result is likely to be.

In the United Kingdom the Law Society may be able to offer names. The Association of Personal Injury Lawyers (APIL) has a brain injury special interest group. The voluntary organization Headway may be able to help. In the United States the American Trial Lawyers Association and State Trial Lawyers Associations can be contacted, and the National Head Injury Foundation will be able to provide information on attorneys specializing in mild head injury litigation.

Having obtained the name of a qualified lawyer in this way it is still necessary to arrange a trial interview with them to make sure that they are in fact interested and adept in the particular area of mild head injury and that they will pursue the case with enthusiasm.

Most people, as consumers, have some skill in evaluating and purchasing such things as cars, refrigerators, and houses, but are often at a loss when it comes to hiring professionals such as lawyers – or doctors. It is necessary to emphasize that as consumers of legal services the client has the absolute right in the initial interview to ask the lawyer various questions about their background and practice in the field of head injury.

At this preliminary interview then it will be reasonable to ask the lawyer questions of the following sort.

(1) How many cases like mine have you been involved in as the principal over the past three years?

(2) What percentage of your practice of law is devoted to cases and injuries like mine?

(3) What were the results in terms of settlements or verdicts for the last five cases that you handled involving cases like mine?

(4) In the last two years have you attended seminars or conferences which involved discussion of injuries such as mine?

(5) Please give the names of three textbooks that you own and consult when seeking information on injuries like mine.

(6) What experts do you expect to be engaging to assist you in the analysis and presentation of my case?

In the long run the lawyer and his or her staff are likely to see more of the patient and especially their family than anyone else, and as well as obtaining satisfactory answers to these questions it is important that there should be an empathy between them.

Opening moves

The lawyer chosen will explore the circumstances of the accident, sometimes with the advice of a traffic engineer and other specialists. They will
often work through a case manager, someone who has expert knowledge
of the information needed and the resources available. They will obtain
detailed information about the patient's past, including school records,
employment and financial status, and an assessment of the current state
and impairment.

First assessment

This will consist of the following parts.

(1) A detailed account from the patient of their symptoms and the way
    in which their daily life is affected.

(2) A neurological assessment, with particular attention to the sense of
    smell, vision, hearing, and balance (see Chapter 6).

(3) A neuropsychological assessment (see Chapter 8).

(4) An account from one, or if possible several, family members and close
    associates, of the patient's performance and apparent symptoms. This
    may differ substantially from the patient's own account, particularly
    if frontal lobe function has been impaired.

(5) Information about the patient's performance before the accident,
    again from close associates but also from documentary records such
    as school and academic grades, employment, with promotions, and
    any other material which seems relevant.

(6) An estimate from the team dealing with the patient's rehabilitation of
    the costs incurred so far and the likely duration of future treatment
    and its cost.

(7) With this information an estimate can be made of the likely degree of
    disability, including earning capacity, and the costs to date, which
    will be the basis of the claim.

Issues which may come up in court – was there a head injury?

In most cases there will be evidence from bystanders, paramedics, or
primary care doctors that there was a loss of consciousness, and this will
be supported by the findings of bruises and other physical evidence of
injury. In a significant minority, however, patients themselves may have

been unaware of a break in the sequence of events, or onlookers may say that they seemed to be awake throughout. This is often the case in vehicular rear end collisions with a whiplash type of injury.

In court the defence lawyers may make much of this and argue that without loss of consciousness any impairment demonstrated is due to other causes. There is, however, good biomedical evidence that rear end collisions at low speeds of the order of 10–15 m.p.h. can result in substantial accelerations to the brain, of the order of 15 g, and that this is sufficient to cause axonal injury and surface damage to the cortex. Also that damage of this sort can occur without the brainstem centres concerned with consciousness being affected. As we pointed out in Chapters 3 and 5, loss of consciousness and later cognitive and behavioural changes do not necessarily march together.

Issues which may come up in court – interpreting neurospychological assessments

The parts of the neurospychological test performance which are typical of head injury are described in Chapter 8, together with the indications that a subject may not be performing as well as they could, or perhaps malingering. In some cases, however, though the history of the accident and the symptoms may be typical, the test results do not follow the usual pattern. This is liable to happen in people who are high achievers. Their scores in most areas may be within normal limits; the reduction in a few critical areas has been sufficient to affect their overall performance. Again, the contribution of fatigue must be taken into account. If the patient is examined when they are fresh their performance may be satisfactory, but it is important also to see them when they are tired, when performance is likely to deteriorate rapidly as the test session proceeds.

It is necessary in presenting the results of neuropsychological testing to relate them to the problems that the patient complains of, and to the problems that are observed by people who knew them both before and after the injury. It is not expected that there will be a perfect fit between these descriptions, but if there is a great disparity one should begin to look for or suspect something other than traumatic brain injury. The issue of the detection of frank malingering is considered in Chapter 8.

Issues which may come up in court – post-traumatic stress disorder

We have discussed this in Chapter 11. Symptoms of PTSD may be playing a significant part in the claimant's disability. It is probable that this syndrome is more likely to occur when the subject has a history of psychiatric disorder, other stressful events in their life, or is a woman. On this account the defendant may claim that the accident has a less responsibility for the claimant's state. In court this argument can only be taken as a diversion. The essence of the situation is that there are neuropsychological deficits, with a substantial and continued change in the capacity for work and family relations. Whatever the theory of the origins of the disability it is the occurrence as a result of the accident that is relevant.

Issues which may come up in court – use of the AMA guides to impairment

The American Medical Association has sponsored the production of successive editions of *Guides to the assessment of permanent impairment* for use in medicolegal work. It examines the consequences of disease and injury of each of the body systems, grades them, and ascribes a percentage of 'impairment of the whole person'. Unfortunately the section on the nervous system, certainly in the last available fourth edition, is misleading when it comes to the assessment of the consequences of mild head injury. It directs that the performance in the workplace is *not* to be taken into consideration, though we know that in many cases the impairment may only show up under the stress of work. It lists five major categories of impairment, of which two are 'mental status' and 'emotional or behavioural', but states that the impairment in only one of these is to contribute to the assessment. In fact both have a significant effect and each must be taken into account.

In the assessment of head injury the *Guide* recommends that the section on mental and behavioural disorders is consulted. However, in this section it is stated that the performance at work *does* need to be taken into account. The general tenor of the section is more appropriate, but the assessment of head injury impairment is not specifically dealt with, and it is difficult to place such a patient in the grades which are appropriate for other mental and behavioural disorders.

For these reasons assessments using the *Guides* are likely substantially to underestimate the patient's disability, and the lawyer must be prepared to counter this with the evidence from the neuropsychologist and those who have been in a position to observe the patient before and after the injury.

Issues which may come up in court – the status of the treating physician

Most readers of this book are likely to be members of the team treating the patient, and their contribution will be the provision of clinical data and some opinions for the use of the lawyer and their case manager. If they appear in court it will be in the first place as a witness of fact. The strength of their evidence will be the opportunity they have had to follow the progress of the patient, and a weakness will be that it is difficult for a good therapist to remain at arms length from their patient. Any answer that they give should, as far as possible, be testimony that could be presented unchanged for use either by the claimant or the defendant. They may also be asked for opinions on cause, on any other assessments that have been produced and on the claimant's future. They should be cautious in answering questions of this sort unless they are familiar with court procedure and are prepared for cross-examination. If they are likely to be in this position, often they would be well advised to attend one of the courses that are available on the skills needed by the expert witness.

In most cases the lawyers on either side will use witnesses not connected with treatment who will qualify as experts and will be expected to produce such opinions. They will need to present credentials showing that they have extensive training and experience in areas relevant to the case being tried, and may expect to be challenged on their competence.

The Court's assessment of disability

The next step, the formal assessment of disability, is the function of the Court. It will be based on the estimate of impairment and on the many factors of the patient's past and future life.

At this stage the detailed account of the claimant's circumstances and everyday activities can be matched with the estimates made of the degree of impairment. There may be evidence of a change of character, perhaps from an outgoing and competent person to someone unsure of themselves, slow on the uptake. They may have just been able to cope with their old job, but were unable to learn a new one. Family will often be able to record difficulty with organizing and everyday activities. They may be able to illustrate this by citing problems such as planning a meal or selecting the clothes appropriate to a particular activity.

The award

The verdict and the amount of the award will be decided on a variety of factors such as culpability and any contribution to the accident by the claimant. Medical and rehabilitation staff will contribute by providing an opinion of the needs and capability of the claimant in the future, with the amount being determined with the help of economic analysts and life-care planners.

Mild head injury litigation – the lawyer's point of view

The lawyer who is retained in a case of mild head injury should base his or her conduct of the case on three principles:

(1) that mild head injury can be serious and significant for the injured person;
(2) that though their head injury has been labelled as mild, the person can experience severe economic consequences such as complete employment disability, together with depression and other problems;
(3) that mild cognitive impairment in areas such as memory, problem solving, attention and concentration, and word retrieval can have a significant and serious impact on the quality of life.

With this in mind, the lawyer should have three main aims, all in keeping with the highest standards of the profession:

(1) to get the injured person adequate, proper, and fair compensation to make up for what they have lost and will lose in the future;
(2) to use their skill and persuasiveness to help and encourage the injured person to obtain appropriate and complete medical care and therapy so that they can get the best quality of life possible;
(3) to detect and weed out fraudulent or over-blown claims.

Though the lawyer should be able to interact at all stages with the injured person and their management, this will generally be as an observer. They are in a sensitive situation, however, as the injured person may find it easier to talk to them and air their problems than to take them to the specialist treating them.

In spite of this the lawyer may have some advantage over the members of the health team. They and their staff may have more time to spend with the injured person and particularly with their family. The information and records that they obtain to establish the past circumstances and performance of the injured person will be of value to the health team, who may not have been in a position to obtain this information.

An important function, which should be a continual care of the lawyer, is to minimize the impact of the litigation on the injured person and not to allow them to be overly focused on it. They should be encouraged to concentrate on getting better and leave the legal aspects to their lawyer.

Lawyers are often faced with difficult, embarrassing, and sometimes insoluble problems. They may recognize that a client who has consulted them about an accident claim has signs and symptoms of a traumatic brain injury, but this has not yet been medically diagnosed. It may be difficult to decide whether to suggest the diagnosis or to adopt a wait-and-see policy, with the risk of their condition worsening with the delay. The lawyer should always remember that they are not a health care provider and they should never suggest a possible diagnosis, though they may recommend that their client should be evaluated by a specialist. In doing this, they can simply tell the client that before they can make any decision what to do on their behalf that there is a type of doctor, maybe a neuropsychologist, who can examine them at their request. The lawyer can then send the information that they have to the specialist and let them make the evaluation and diagnosis and discuss this with the injured person.

It is strongly recommended that the lawyer should not get involved in the medical diagnosis, showing pictures of the brain or explaining how injury affects it; this can make the injured person's complaints seem contrived and compromise a legitimate claim for damages.

Nevertheless, in some circumstances it may be difficult for the lawyer not to intervene in medical management. An instance is when strong pressure is put on the injured person to return to work when the lawyer knows that the effort will be unsuccessful and that this will result in further emotional suffering. In issues of this sort the lawyer must be painfully aware that their motives are always suspect. However, as the guardian of the client's interests they may be obliged to take action.

Mild head injuries under a no-fault compensation system

In 1974 New Zealand introduced a no-fault compensation system for personal injury by accident, the Accident Compensation Commission (ACC). At the same time the right to sue for damages was abolished. Eighty per cent of wages were paid from the time of the accident if it occurred at work, or after a week for other accidents; this payment continued until return to work was possible. If they could not earn as much as before the accident because of a disability, 80 per cent of the difference was made up. Medical treatment and rehabilitation were provided by the state health system; if there was delay in obtaining this, part of the costs of private treatment might be covered. If there was a permanent disability, the impairment was estimated and a lump sum payment proportional to this was made; there was also a lump sum payment for loss of enjoyment of life. Entry to the scheme was by a medical certificate from the medical practitioner responsible for the initial treatment, which was renewed by GPs or specialists as required by the patient's condition. Case managers oversaw administration details and gave help with arranging rehabilitation facilities.

The system had great advantages. Family income, though uncomfortably reduced, was still maintained at a level which avoided hardship. Rehabilitation and resettlement in work could be done deliberately. The administrative costs were very much less than those of litigation. However, injured people with a long term disability were often dissatisfied by the amount of the lump sum payment, though they generally failed to take into account that their salary compensation payments would continue for the rest of their lives and amount to many times the lump sum.

Subsequent governments have modified the scheme, largely because of perceptions of abuse and also because of a change in political principles. In 1992 the lump sums were abolished and a system of regular payments based on an estimate of disability was instituted. With the frequent changes in regulations demanded by parliament, the administration has become over-complex and some, but by no mean all, of the advantages have been lost.

The great majority of people who suffer a mild head injury have only a short contact with the ACC. In most cases the initial certificate of injury will be filled out but in many the period of disability will be no more than a few days and nothing more will be done. When they are likely to be off work for ten days or more, most will apply for weekly payments. Where there is a continuing disability this immediate support is valuable because it relieves much of the anxiety about finance which can hinder progress.

A major problem in systems such as this, experienced in New Zealand and elsewhere, is that a small proportion of patients can prolong the period of their disability; this occurs particularly when the injury occurred at work. A well organized rehabilitation service will minimize the incidence, but in many places this facility is not available and the insurer may depend on certificates from doctors without the means or experience to deal with the problem.

To deal with this problem the ACC has recently instituted regular assessments by a medical panel independent of the treating physician. Unfortunately the act of parliament which governs the ACC specifies that impairment is to be estimated with the help of the AMA *Guides to the evaluation of impairment*. As explained above, these are not reliable when used for head injury, particularly mild injury. This was a major problem when it was necessary to assess patients for lump sum payments, and remains when used for the periodical assessments.

However, in spite of the problems that have affected it, the no-fault principle has much to recommend it.

Further reading

Braithwaite, W. (1996). Legal considerations. In *Brain injury and after: towards improved outcome*, (ed. F. D. Rose and D. A. Johnson). Wiley, Chichester.
This is a useful guide to the subject from the United Kingdom point of view.
Simkins, C. N. (ed.) (1994). *Analysis, understanding and presentation of cases involving traumatic brain injury.* National Head Injury Foundation, 1776 Massachusetts Avenue, NW, Suite 100, Washington DC 20036, USA.
This large, loose-leaf volume – 600 pages – is an encyclopaedic reference dealing with clinical features of the problems following head injuries, their rehabilitation, and the considerations of legal representation.

Appendices

Contents

1. Orientation and memory scales

These were referred to in Chapter 4 and provide convenient tests.

2. Precautions for patients allowed home from emergency departments

Most emergency departments will have their own handouts; this may be a useful supplement or basis for others to prepare their own material.

3. Policy for management of concussion sustained at school

We have found that in many schools the teaching staff may not be well informed about the immediate and long term effects of milder head injury. This paper was prepared at the request of nurses working at schools, for their own guidance and for that of the teaching staff.

4. Advice for people who have had a mild head injury or who have been concussed

Most people who have had minimal head injuries will find that the discharge sheet given in Appendix 2 will give them enough information. For others who have had rather more severe injuries, who may be relatively isolated after discharge or who seem to wish for more detailed information, it is useful to have a more substantial handout.

5. Getting back to work at the desk

Professional and business people and students at school and university have special problems in getting back to work. We have found that a supplement to face to face consultation is useful, both as a means of refreshing their memory of what we have told them and as something to show family and possibly employers and fellow workers.

6. Rivermead symptom checklist

This is a well validated symptom checklist for patients to fill in themselves. Its use is mentioned in Chapter 5.

7. Glasgow Coma Scale for children

There are several modified scores suitable for children; this one is relatively simple and practical.

Acknowledgements

Appendices 1 and 2 were prepared by the authors for use in their own hospital. Appendix 3 was prepared at the request of school nurses.

Appendices 4 and 5 have been modified from the texts of booklets which the authors prepared for the New Zealand Neurological Foundation. The Foundation holds the copyright, but is happy for the text to be used without obtaining formal permission, though it would appreciate acknowledgement of the source.

Appendix 6, the Rivermead PCS Questionnaire, is reprinted from King, N. S. Emotional, neuropsychological and organic factors: their use in the prediction of persisting postconcussion symptoms after moderate and mild head injuries. (1996) *Journal of Neurology, Neurosurgery, and Psychiatry*, **61**, 75–81. This again may reproduced freely, but the source should be acknowledged.

Appendix 7 is reproduced by courtesy of the Trauma Service of the Starship Children's Hospital, Auckland, and may be used with acknowledgement.

Appendix 1
Orientation and memory scales

Orientation

Questions

1. What is your name	0	1	2
2. Where do you live?	0	1	2
3. When is your birthday?	0	1	2
How old are you?	0	1	
4. Where are you now?	0		2
5. Which hospital?	0		2
6. Which department?	0		2
7. What day of the week today?	0	1	2
8. What month is it now?	0	1	2
9. What year is it now?	0	1	
10. What happened to you?	0	1	2

Possible total	20
Controls	17 or over

Notes on scoring

- The correct answer scores 2, except questions 3 and 9.
- An answer that is definitely wrong, or no answer, scores 0.
- If the answer is not correct but close to it, it may be scored 1.
- If the answer is correct but takes a long time or needs prompting, score 1.

Using these criteria a group of ED trauma patients who had not had head injuries were given the test. All scores 17 or over. The questions on which controls most often failed were 'What department?' and 'Where are you now?', which may be difficult for people unfamiliar with hospitals.

Memory

The patient is given the names of two everyday objects to remember. They are tested after 15 minutes; if they can recall both objects continuous memory has returned. If they cannot, the test is repeated.

Remember – orientation and memory may not return together; a patient can be oriented and amnesic or confused and remember.

Note: These two are simple tests for use when the patient presents in the ED. They are not sufficiently searching for later use.

Appendix 2
Precautions for patients
allowed home

Instructions and important precautions for people who have had a mild head injury and who are well enough to return home after treatment in the emergency department

The first 24 h

For the patient

You have had an injury to your head with concussion. The doctors have examined you and have found that there has been no serious damage. It is safe for you to go home now, but in the next 24 h there could still be changes in your condition which need treatment.

The people who are with you have been asked to watch you and to make sure you come back to hospital if you are not well.

After a few days you will probably feel that you are getting back to normal. On the back of this sheet there are suggestions what you should then do about driving, going back to work, or playing sport.

For the relatives or friends

Though it is unlikely, it is possible that in the next 24 h the patient could develop serious complications that would need urgent hospital treatment. If this was happening, you might find that they would:

- become drowsy or actually lose consciousness
- sleep so deeply that you could not wake them
- have a severe and continuous headache
- vomit repeatedly.

If this happens, take them back to hospital. If they seem to be losing consciousness this is **urgent** and no time should be lost.

If they leave hospital in the evening, over the first night you should wake them at least twice to make sure that they are not developing complications.

Stitches

Stitches have been put in. These should be removed in . . . days.

Pain relief

Headache is common after concussion. You may take paracetamol (*local name*) or similar pills, but should avoid any which contain aspirin in any of its forms. If the headache is severe, you should see the doctor.

After 24 h

After 24 h serious complications can still occur, but are much less likely.

Though your injury has not been severe, probably you will not feel that you have completely recovered for ten days or so.

It is common to have a headache for two or three days, and this may be worse with exercise. You may feel unsteady or giddy.

Many people find it difficult to concentrate for the first few days, and cannot work out problems as easily as usual. They may find themselves getting bad tempered and irritable.

After four or five days most people are very much better. If you do not think that you are completely right by 14 days after the accident you should see your family doctor or return to this department.

Driving

It will be unsafe for you to drive for at least 24 h after the accident. You may be slow to react for several more days and you should not start to drive again until you are quite free of symptoms. Then, start with caution and avoid long trips or heavy traffic.

Work

If you don't feel your normal self and cannot concentrate you are unlikely to be much use at work, and it is better to stay off for a few days. If it is possible, it is better to start by working part time for a day or two, until you have got back into the swing. Most young people can expect to be back to normal work after 10 days.

Sport

Ordinary exercise can start when headache, tiredness, or dizziness allow it. Contact sports where another concussion is possible should not be played for three weeks – for some sports bodies this time off play is compulsory.

If at any time you feel you are not making a proper recovery, come back to this department or see your family doctor.

(Prepared by authors)

Appendix 3
Concussion sustained at school

Pupils can be concussed by falls in the school buildings or play areas, and in organized games. Almost all will recover quickly, but occasionally there are complications, both immediately after the injury and when the pupil is well enough to return to school. These may be serious and it is important that there should be a school policy for dealing with concussion and that all staff members should be aware of it.

Decisions needed at the time of the accident

Has the pupil been concussed?

Symptoms of concussion

From the pupil:

- says that they were 'out' or unaware of what was going on for a period, however short;
- headache that is more than mild soreness, nausea, dizziness.

From others:

- a period of unresponsiveness, however short – did not open eyes, speak, or get up at once;
- confusion – didn't know what to do, how to play, even for a moment;
- unsteadiness – unable to keep balance.

Tests of normality

- Balance – should be able to stand straight up without swaying, and to walk heel-to-toe steadily.
- Orientation – must be able to give their name and address, age, day of the week, where they are.
- Memory – should remember how the accident occurred, what happened afterwards.

If they describe *any* of the symptoms above, or if they cannot pass *all* the tests of normality, it must be taken that they have been concussed. It is *not* necessary for there to have been a loss of consciousness obvious to bystanders.

What action should be taken if a pupil has been concussed?

By school staff

If they are still unconscious, drowsy, or confused, staff should arrange for them to be taken to a doctor immediately, preferably to hospital.

Recommendation to parents

If there is no doubt that they have been unconscious but now seem to have recovered completely, they should be seen by a doctor that day.

If there has been no observed loss of consciousness but any of the other symptoms described above, the pupil should be seen by a doctor within a day or two to make sure there are no persisting problems.

On return to school

Poor performance

Class teachers should be aware that people who have been concussed, even slightly, will often at first have some or all of the following set of symptoms.

- Difficulty in concentrating, and so of keeping up with class work.
- Tiring easily, and getting a headache when they are tired.
- Performance falling off quickly when they are tired.
- Short temper, irritability, and in severe cases disruptive behaviour.

In most cases, if they occur, these symptoms will clear in a week or so. However, often after more severe injuries and occasionally after lesser ones, the symptoms will persist.

There is a danger that the symptoms can be confused with the behaviour of the pupil who is choosing not to work at school, and that this will be taken to be the cause.

It is important therefore that when school work and behaviour seem to have deteriorated after a head injury, a proper diagnosis is made. If head injury is the cause a special management programme will be needed to avoid long term effects.

If it is suspected that deterioration of school work and behaviour is due to a head injury, a medical check and neuropsychological testing will be needed.

Playing sport again

Someone who has been concussed, however quickly they seem to recover, should not go back on the field and continue to play. After concussion people are often less coordinated and their reaction times are slower, so that further injury is more likely.

After a definite concussion, contact sport should not be resumed for at least three weeks. A second head injury within this period, even if it is a minor one, can have serious or fatal results.

If later, after the three week period, a pupil has a second concussion, they should not play again that season. If in the next season they have another concussion they should consider changing to a non-contact sport.

Young people need their maximum brain capacity to learn and make their way in life, and it is wise to be even more cautious than these re-commendations about continuing contact sports.

Appendix 4
Advice for the patient

Advice for people who have had a mild head injury and have been concussed

If you are reading this it's likely that you have had a mild head injury yourself or that you are close to someone who has. We hope it will help you to understand what has happened and to deal with the problems that may follow.

Most of us are familiar with the typical story of someone who gets concussed. They are knocked out playing football and wake up at the side of the field dazed and confused. They are taken to the emergency department at the local hospital and after an hour or two they are well enough to go home. They feel bad for 24 h, go back to work a day or two later, and in a month have almost forgotten the whole incident.

Unfortunately this isn't the complete picture. Some people have unpleasant symptoms for several weeks after being concussed, and in a few of them the problems can last much longer.

Most people who have had this happen to them are not aware of this, and they may become very concerned, anxious, and sometimes depressed. They may be afraid they have 'brain damage' or that they will never be back to normal. They may make wrong decisions about their future, and can lose the sympathy and understanding of their family and friends.

The good news is that these unpleasant symptoms don't last for ever, and that if they are properly managed there should be no serious long-term effects. What follows will tell you what may happen and what to do about it.

The first two weeks

Most people who have been concussed won't feel that they are completely back to normal again until after a fortnight or so. Here are some of the things that may worry you, and what to do about them.

Tiredness

Your brain will seem to have less energy. After even a little effort you may feel worn out and be unable to go on. You will want to go to bed early and sleep longer.

When you feel like this, don't feel ashamed to rest or go to bed. Your brain is telling you that you need to rest – listen to it. If you struggle on, you will only make yourself even more tired and less able to cope.

Poor concentration

Concentration depends on being alert, and it's the first thing to fail when you get tired. If you are tired and can't concentrate, rest. If there's something you must get done, start when you have had a sleep and are feeling fresh, and then stop as soon as your attention begins to fade. If you haven't finished, have a rest and then try again.

Forgetting things

You may forget where you put your glasses or what you went to the shops for, but can remember as well as ever what happened a year ago. This is partly because you're concentrating badly, but also because concussion puts the memory system out of order for a while. Don't be alarmed, it will get better. Meanwhile, concentrate when there is something which you want to remember, and if it is important, make a note of it – it won't stop your memory recovering.

Irritability

Often people who have been concussed find that they easily get annoyed by things that normally wouldn't worry them. They lose their temper for nothing, snap at their family or their workmates, and perhaps get themselves into trouble because of it. This happens because self-control, like concentrating and remembering, needs a brain that's fresh and working well.

The first thing to do is to be on the watch for it happening. If you feel your irritation is going to burst out, turn away, go out of the room, take time out. Relieve your tension by learning ways to relax – we'll mention this later – or use up your aggression by taking exercise or hitting a punch-bag.

Noise

Putting up with noise needs brain energy, and people find it difficult after they have been concussed. Children playing, a loud radio, or machinery at work may be unbearable. The only remedy is to avoid the noise – ask the family to help you by turning the volume down, get the grandparents to take the children for a day or two, or buy some ear protectors.

Dizziness

Concussion sometimes upsets the balance organs in the ears, and for a short while after the injury a sudden movement of your head can give you vertigo, so that the world seems to spin round you. More often people have a feeling of unreality or floating, which they describe as dizziness. Both these settle down in time, but can be disturbing if you are not prepared for them.

Clumsiness

When you are recovering from concussion you may find that you bump into people in the street, or drop the dishes when you're drying them. Again, this is your brain reacting more slowly and being less efficient than usual. Take it as a warning that you should take special care when there could be danger, like crossing the street, and of course you shouldn't be driving your car if you are reacting slowly.

Eye problems

After concussion people often find that bright light worries them, and that it helps to wear sunglasses, even indoors. Sight is sometimes a little blurred, either because the eyes are not focusing well, or because they are not lining up correctly. Again this is the result of the brain not working as well as usual. This almost always comes right of its own, but get expert advice if it doesn't get better.

Headache

Headaches can be expected in the early stages because of the bruising from the injury. Later they are often due to tiredness and stress, when you are asking your brain to do more than it is capable of. This sort of headache can usually be relieved by resting, and prevented by making sure you stop work as soon as you feel tired. Headache pills often don't make much difference to this sort of pain. If it becomes severe and will not go away you should see your doctor.

What to do if the symptoms don't go away

Most people will have at least some of these symptoms after they have been concussed, but they should be almost free of them by a fortnight.

However, about one person in ten will take longer to recover. If your symptoms have lasted for more than two or three weeks, or are particularly severe, you should ask for professional help.

The first thing that will be done is make sure that there are none of the unlikely but serious complications of the injury. Then probably tests will be made of concentration and memory, the way the brain is working, to serve as a guide to treatment, and as a baseline to measure progress.

Once there is no doubt about the cause, you can be reassured that the symptoms will eventually clear, even though it may take a little time. The problems that have to be tackled are the misery they cause while they last, and the upset of family life, job, and earning power that results.

Organizing help

How this is done will depend on what's available where you live. A good option is a team with a doctor, psychologist, occupational therapist, and social worker, and this may be available at your local hospital or clinic. They will be able to begin treatment and to talk to you and your family, and perhaps arrange a meeting with other people with the same problems.

Once it is clear what the problems are, a programme can be worked out. Often the first things to fix are money and family problems. They are important causes of anxiety and stress, and because of poor concentration and lack of energy they may have not been dealt with properly. The social worker will be able to help with this.

When the symptoms of concussion have not cleared in two or three weeks you could become quite anxious and depressed, and an important part of the programme would be to help you to get over this. To begin with, either by yourself or with one of your family, you would need to talk to a member of the team who could explain the problems and how they could be tackled. Often, because you might not be taking things in well, this might have to be gone through several times. As well as this, it's often helpful to have a talk to other people who have had the same problems. If you found that worry was getting the better of you, the team might arrange for you to learn relaxation exercises and have special help with stress management.

A daily routine

Having a well planned daily routine is an important part of treatment, and the team should help you to work one out. If you are not concentrating and are tired and irritable you should be off work to begin with, but you still need a regular programme of things to do, both brain work and physical. This has to be enough to make you feel that you have achieved something, but it must not make you more than a little tired. The essential parts of the programme are listed below.

Rest

You must learn to pace yourself and rest when you are tired, and you must never get so tired that you don't feel fresh again after a night's rest.

Increase gradually

As you get better you should only slowly step up the amount you do, each time making sure that you can cope with what you are doing before you make a change.

Get back to work by easy stages

As you can find you can do more and more, you can think of starting work again. It is important that you take the return to work in easy stages. The ideal is to start with working just half a day, three days a week, and then to increase the time at work slowly, only when it's certain that you can cope and that fatigue will not build up from day to day. This of course depends on your job and your employer, and the team may be able to help in setting up a practical programme.

Get people to understand

It's important that others know what's happening, that the symptoms are real and directly due to the accident. Because most people don't understand what the effects of concussion are, family, friends, workmates, or employer may think that it's all been put on, that 'they could do better if they tried' or 'they just want some time off to lay about at home'.

It can be difficult to convince people. Showing them these pages may help, and the team should be glad to talk to your family, and to your employer.

Getting the help you need

If you have problems after a mild head injury, you should see your doctor to make sure that there are no complications. They may look after you themselves or may prefer to send you to see a neurologist or a neuro-psychologist.

When you have been given a programme of treatment, it's often difficult to follow it on your own. you may be able to go regularly to the hospital or clinic and discuss the problems with the occupational therapist or another counsellor; sometimes home visits can be arranged. It often helps to discuss problems with other people with the same condition, and in many places there will be support groups that you could join.

If there are compensation or legal consequences of your accident, make sure you get help – they should be dealt with as soon as possible and you probably won't be very good at dealing with them yourself until you feel better.

Special problems with mild head injury

Children – pre-school and primary school

This is the time when the brain has most learning to do and a head injury can have a definite effect on a child's progress. Family and teachers may not realize that this can happen. If there is any suggestion that after a head injury, even a mild one, your child is not progressing as well as it should, you should get expert help.

School and university

People at school and university also depend on their ability to learn, and again even a short period of incapacity at a critical time, such as the run-up to an exam, can have a serious effect. They or their families may not want to admit that there is a problem, but if there is a suggestion that they are having unexpected difficulty with their work, they should ask for expert advice.

Older people

As people reach middle age they are likely to be more affected by a head injury. The symptoms they have are the same but they often need more help and more time to get over them.

People who work on their own

Homemakers and people with their own businesses can have special difficulty in managing their head injury symptoms. Often they feel that they can't stop working, and so deny that they're ill. Because they're not coping, the problems mount up and they become more and more stressed until a crisis occurs. Family and friends then need to persuade them to accept help and reduce their work load, and to get expert advice.

Sports injuries – when to play again

Concussion is quite common in some sports, and there may be pressure to play down its effects. It is dangerous to life to risk a second concussion within a week or two of the first one. Some sports bodies have strict rules about this and it is irresponsible not to follow them.

More than one head injury

Each head injury, even mild concussion, results in a slight long term reduction of the capacity of the brain. The reserve of brain power that we all have will compensate for the loss after one or two injuries, but if there are more the loss will start to show, by slowing of thought, poor memory, and change of character. Those who have had more than one injury should think carefully before exposing themselves to repeated risks, such as those of football and boxing. A good rule is not to play again that season if you have had two concussions, and to give up the sport if you have one more.

What you should remember after having a mild head injury

- **Do not** drive your car or motorbike until you have made sure that your concentration is good and your reactions are fast enough.

- **Do not** expect to deal with alcohol in the usual way until you have fully recovered. One small drink may lay you flat.

- **Do not** expose yourself to the risk of another injury. until you have recovered completely. Your reactions will be slow and you may be clumsy, just inviting a second accident.

- **Do not** think it's giving in to have a rest when you are tired. It's not a sin to have a sleep in the afternoon. Do not swear to finish papering the room when you feel tired, even if it kills you. It may.

- **Do** start work again by easy stages, **do not** let your mates pressure you to work longer than you feel you can.

Appendix 5
Back to work 'at the desk'

Foreword

This booklet has been written for people who are trying to get back to their work 'at the desk'. These are people in professions and business, and at school and university.

Yours is the sort of job in which you have to listen to people, to read and take in what you read, to discuss and argue, to sort all this out and then produce answers and make decisions. As well as this you will probably have to be sensitive to the attitudes and body language of the people you're dealing with, and to be aware of what other people in turn are thinking of you.

This is a tall order, because these skills are just the ones that are regularly affected by head injuries, even by mild ones.

Getting over this sort of injury therefore is not easy. If your brain is not yet in good problem solving order, it will be difficult to work out the best way to organize your recovery. If your critical sense has been affected you may not want to accept the help you need.

The people around – family, friends, and employer – may not understand why you're having difficulty. You may hear 'It's six months since the accident so you ought to be right by now' or 'I can't see anything wrong with you', as if they expect your head to be in a bandage if there was.

With all this in mind, the best way we can help is to explain the sorts of problems that you are likely to have and how they arise, and then offer suggestions on how to deal with them.

How a head injury can affect you

Damage to your brain can affect everything you do. It may affect physical activities – hand strength and skills, balance, walking, and running. Here we will be concentrating on the way it affects the way you think.

How bad was the injury? One measure is the length of time after the accident for which you were unconscious, or about which you can't remember anything. More important, though, is the effect it has had on what you can or can't do. In a general way the two measurements go together, so that worse effects follow a longer loss of memory. What many people don't realize is that long term bad effects can also occur after quite mild injuries, like being knocked out at football; it's a matter of luck whether the force of the injury falls on an important part of the brain.

What can you do to put it right? There are no magic cures, but your brain will steadily get better on its own if you give it a chance. It must have practice at doing the things it was good at. It must not be overused or fatigued, and it must not have its energy drained by emotional stress.

We will emphasize again and again that the control of fatigue and stress is the key to managing recovery. It's not easy to achieve this. You desperately want to get back to work, to earning, and to a normal life, and so you push yourself to do more, even if you're tired. You hate being on the shelf, your family is worried, perhaps people don't understand your difficulties, so you're in emotional stress.

To manage this situation you need to understand it, and the next section will help you to do this.

How head injury affects thinking – and what to do about it

The parts of thinking that matter here are concentration, memory, organization, self-control, and fatigue. We'll talk about them separately, though they all interact with each other.

Concentration

Concentration and attention are words which describe how you can keep your mind fixed on what you're doing. It's important because most of the other functions of the brain that we're concerned with depend on it. As an obvious example, if you don't concentrate on what someone is saying, you won't remember what they said. As well as this, concentration is linked to the speed at which you can deal with information and process it.

Concentration is impaired for some time after all head injuries in which consciousness has been lost. It can also be impaired when there has been no loss of consciousness, for example in the 'whiplash' sort of accident.

As part of fixing your mind on the matter in hand, concentration requires you to shut out distractions. If you're not doing this well, you will find that other people's voices, music in the distance, or someone fiddling with a pencil will make you lose concentration, and at the same time probably make you angry and bring on fatigue.

Memory

There are several sorts of memory. Recall of trivial things that have happened in the last hour or two is recent memory. When it is impaired you forget where you put your spectacles, who came to lunch, or what you had to get at the shops. It will be bad if your concentration is poor.

Events that you would expect to remember days or weeks later are stored in long term memory. Things you do repeatedly, either as everyday routine or as part of your professional skills are called 'overlearned' and are firmly fixed in this part of memory.

Head injuries almost always affect memory to some extent. Immediately after the injury, for minutes, hours, or days depending on the severity of the injury, the brain stops recording passing events. Though you may have recovered consciousness and be able to answer quite searching questions about yourself or your surroundings, this is not being stored in your memory – you are in 'post-traumatic amnesia'. When you start recording events again you will find that there is a gap in memory from the moment of the accident; occasionally short 'islands' of memory remain, but the rest never comes back.

It's not surprising that after this period of complete failure memory should take some time to recover. The worst difficulty is with memory for events in the last hour or two or the last day or two. This results in trivial annoyance – where did I put my spectacles – and more serious disability when important information is forgotten and appointments missed.

Longer term memory is also affected, both storing new memories and recalling old ones. Both sorts of memory depend very much on concentration, and recall will be much more difficult when you're tired or surrounded by distractions.

Organization

Some people start the day knowing exactly what they have to do and the order to do it in, and can reorganize if the original plan is upset. Others are less confident, need to think it out and then write a list. After a head injury people are usually even less sure of how to organize themselves and plan their day, and unless they concentrate on what needs doing and write a list, bits will be forgotten. Even then, if anything goes wrong, they fail to cope with the changes needed.

Self-control

Dealing effectively with something that annoys or threatens you needs a brain that functions quickly and efficiently, and which can restrain an instinctive angry or even violent response.

After head injury people find it difficult to cope with the little annoyances of everyday life and tend to snap back; this of course is worse when they are tired.

Insight

To get on with people, at home and at work, you need to be able to look at your own behaviour realistically, and to read other peoples' reactions to you from the subtleties of what they say or their body language. This is a complex and difficult skill, and after head injury may be too much to manage. This can show up as inappropriate behaviour towards others, perhaps undue familiarity or neglecting ordinary social rules.

The other important result of losing insight is that you may become unrealistic about how much your abilities have been affected, and be unwilling to accept advice or warnings.

Fatigue

People normally adjust the amount of work they do each day and the hours they spend in rest and sleep so that the next day they can follow the same pattern without becoming tired enough to affect their efficiency. If there is extra work that just has to be done, they can push themselves to complete it; they may need to go to bed early that night and feel tired next day, but they can carry on in spite of this.

After a head injury the amount of energy that you have is limited. To begin with you may be able to cope with only a few minutes of concentration, either listening, talking, or reading. If you try to press on and do more, the effort is too great, and you soon find you just can't go on. As you recover, longer periods of concentration are possible, but the barrier at the end remains.

If you can live with this, and stop just before you meet the barrier and take a rest, you can often achieve a lot. If you neglect the signals and do more than this, your fatigue will accumulate, a night's sleep won't be enough for you to recover, and next day you will be washed out and good for nothing.

It's like a bank account. You're given so much energy each day; if you overdraw, next day you have less to start with and fatigue comes on earlier. Keep on, and you'll be a wreck by the end of the week.

It is important to keep yourself in as good physical condition as possible. You should find out what sort of physical activity you can manage without overtiring yourself. This could be gardening, walking, or swimming, or a formal exercise programme in a gym if this is what you are used to.

Mood and emotions

It's not easy to get over the effects of head injury, and if progress is slow you may get depressed. Because the injury will have reduced your control over your emotions, you will get upset easily. You may find yourself weeping for not reason. It's important to deal with the depression. Talk it over with your doctor; support, counselling, and sometimes medication will help.

Special problems with thinking

The problems described above are those which almost everyone encounters when they have been affected by head injury. Some people have more specific difficulties with thinking, the common ones being concerned with finding and remembering words, or being able to deal with shapes, sizes, plans, and locations. It is outside the scope of this booklet to get into these in detail; ask the people who are helping with your recovery.

Tests

In the early days after the injury medical examinations are geared to making sure that there are no complications of the injury, such as blood clots pressing on the brain. A CT scan may be needed at this stage.

As you get better, the important thing becomes the way your brain is working, and at this stage special tests of thinking are useful. Measuring your power of concentration and the speed at which you can deal with information is probably the best overall test of function, and a good guide to when you're ready to start with some work. Tests of your ability to organize are also useful for this. In the early stages screening tests may be done to see if you have any of the special problems in thinking that were mentioned above.

Getting on with rehabilitation

When you have recovered from the early effects of the injury, it is time to think of the ways you can prepare to get back to work.

People to consult

It's important that you should have someone to advise you about this first stage of your recovery. Who can do this depends on what's available where you are. Sources of help are your family doctor, the occupational therapy department at your local hospital, or special head injury services that may be available in larger centres. What follows will help you to make some of the arrangements for yourself, and supplement what others have suggested.

A programme

When the worst effects of the accident have settled and you can start doing things around the house with reasonable comfort, it's essential to work out a programme and stick to it. It's so easy to get into the habit of an aimless day, and difficult to get out of it when it's time to start back to work. It's even more difficult after a head injury, because, as we said before, planning and organizing ability are often affected.

A timetable

The first thing to do is to write a timetable. Put down the time you get up in the morning, when you have your breakfast and other meals as fixed points. Early in the day, when you're fresh, put down a time for some activity connected with your work – reading, writing, or making things with your hands. To begin with this will only last for a very short time, perhaps half an hour, because it will tire you.

Make a commitment to a time for exercise. As we said above, most people find that though thinking is tiring, a reasonable amount of exercise is not. Walking is good to start with (it's helpful if you have a dog). Later on a more formal programme may be helpful.

What is vital is that you must rest as soon as you feel tired, and rest for long enough so that the tiredness doesn't accumulate.

Making a timetable like this may not be easy for you. It may be difficult to be realistic about what you can do. Discuss it with the person who is advising you about your recovery and make sure you're on the right track.

Other programmes

If your doctor can arrange for time at an occupational therapy department or at a head injury centre you will be able to join in their programme. This will probably help you to get better more quickly, as well as relieving the boredom of being alone at home, unwell, and without your usual work.

Support groups

Many people find it's useful to be able to discuss problems and exchange solutions with other people with the same problem, and there may be support groups in your area that you could attend.

Steps in returning to work

Are you ready?

Have you tried doing some work at home? If this is not practical, have you tried applying yourself to some other job which needs concentration? When you can do this at a reasonable pace for one and a half or two hours, you may be ready to try back at your ordinary work.

How do you get on with talking to people outside the immediate family? Can you keep up a conversation for ten minutes without feeling frustrated or tired?

The tests mentioned that we described earlier will help to decide, especially those that focus on concentration and speed of reaction.

Do you need to drive at the job, or getting there and back? If you do, reaction times when you are tested should first be within safe limits, and then, if there is any doubt, you should have a driving assessment by a professional instructor.

Planning the return to work

Everyone is different, and the plan needs to be geared to the severity of the symptoms, the sort of work you do, and the support that's available. It will usually be best worked out with the team concerned with your rehabilitation, and then discussed with your prospective employer. This may be the person you worked for before, or it may be better to start with someone who is more able to accommodate any special arrangements that are needed before you are back to your former capacity.

As a general rule it's better to leave return to work until you're fairly sure that you'll be able to cope; most employers will be cooperative if you can stay with the plan proposed, but may get restless if you find you have to reduce the hours that were proposed or take more time off.

A good way of starting back is to begin with a very short period at work, two hours a day is often about right, on three days a week. Mondays, Wednesdays, and Fridays are best, so that there is a day to rest after each day at work. This can then be increased slowly, to begin with by not more than half an hour a day each week, making sure that there is no undue fatigue and that at the end of the week you don't feel tired out. When you can manage four hours three times a week, do an extra day, perhaps starting with only two hours that day, and working up. Carry on like that, always being sure that you don't become so tired that the fatigue accumulates and lasts until the next day. A programme of this sort may sound very slow and over-cautious. In your case you may be able to speed it up, but if you try to do this be doubly careful to watch for the signs of accumulating fatigue, and remember that an unexpected problem or even a late night can set you back.

Remember that it's impossible to say how long it will take before you're back to normal working hours, and it's not a good idea to make prophecies, because if they don't work out – and they can never be more than guesses – you will be discouraged and may lose heart.

Some people will find that they have to accept a long term reduction in the time they can work for. Their productivity in the hours they are able to work may be good, and up to their old standard, but they may continue having to go home one or two hours earlier each day, if they are to avoid getting progressively more tired.

Even though you are making sure that you don't get too tired at work, you may find that when the weekend comes you only want to sleep most of the time and don't have energy for family or social activities. This is tough on the family and friends, and the family particularly should be told before you return to work that this is something that may well happen.

Special needs

Primary school children

Concentration, memory, and learning new skills are vital in primary school, but are just the abilities that are affected by head injury. Again, like adults, head injured children tire quickly and their capacity falls off. Problems in behaviour show up as well; the children are easily distracted, distract others, and can become disruptive in class.

Good relations with an understanding principal and teachers are needed. It should be agreed that the child starts back with very limited hours, perhaps only one or two periods a day, and then increases the time by small amounts only when they are able to cope comfortably. It's desirable that there should be a quiet area where the child can go to if they are getting tired or disruptive, or arrangements for them to go back home if this occurs. To begin with, an afternoon sleep may be needed.

It will often be impossible for the class teacher to give enough time to the child to help them to catch up and keep up with the others in the class. Time with a special teacher may be needed; for how long each week will depend on how much it adds to the child's tiredness.

Secondary

The basic problems and solutions are the same as those of return to primary school, but managing them may be more difficult. The pressures to succeed are tougher. Several teachers for different subjects are involved and it may be difficult to have them all aware of the problems and to make the allowances needed. Later on there are critical exams to sit. Adolescence creates its own problems and stresses, which make recovery more difficult. It may be necessary to work hard with principals, deans, and teachers to get the care that's needed.

University

University courses demand drive and organization as well as concentration and memory – all abilities that will be impaired after head injury. Even more than in other occupations, you will need to have a realistic and attainable programme for return to work. You and the rehabilitation team should work this out with the tutors and faculty members responsible, remembering that if your insight is impaired you may think that you are capable of much more than you really can cope with.

With this programme you may be able to cope with term work and assignments quite well, but may fail in exams because of the stress and time limitation. If you think this is likely to happen, tell your tutor; extra writing time will usually be allowed.

Making these adjustments, with the financial and social stresses which will follow them, may be as much as you can cope with, and you will need all the support you can get from family, friends, and rehabilitation people.

The self-employed

If you have your own business you will face the problems both of finding ways to keep the business going while you are disabled, and then of taking over the work again by easy stages as you recover. It's unfortunately common to find that the need to keep the business going will force people to try to do their usual work when they are not capable of it. This creates more stress, performance deteriorates further, and a crisis situation develops. The business can be damaged, and you can be pushed into a serious loss of confidence and breakdown as a result.

In this situation, you need good counselling to begin with, so that you can accept the impairment that has resulted from the head injury. This is often difficult, both because of concern about the survival of the business and because your insight and judgement may have been affected by the injury. You then need a realistic plan of action. You need to get support from people with appropriate skills that can help you to keep the business going. When you can take some work up again, you must again accept advice to make sure that it is within your capacity and that fatigue and stress don't accumulate.

Administrators and professionals

As we said in the introduction, this is the sort of job in which you have to listen to people, to read and take in what you read, to discuss and argue, and then to sort all this out, produce answers, and make decisions. As we have seen, all these activities can be affected by head injury, and all result in, and are sensitive to, fatigue.

When you go back to work, then, like the other groups you should start with restricted hours. You should arrange it so that you only work until you first begin to be tired, and then either go home or have a substantial rest before starting work again.

Make a list of the things you have to do in order of their importance. Do the essentials that make most of your special skills, and delegate as much of the other work as you can to others. Do one thing at a time – switching jobs takes a lot of energy.

The difficult work should be done first thing in the day when you are fresh. Most people find that meetings are difficult to cope with – following the argument round the table and concentrating on what people are saying – so try to schedule these for the morning.

Resuming work after an interruption is more difficult after a head injury. When you have a task to do, turn off your telephone, or have people call you only in an emergency.

Have a rest in the middle of the day, with absolutely no interruptions. Use stress management techniques (the occupational therapists, and others, can teach you these) or learn to meditate.

Days will come when after lunch you will feel fine, and able to get through a mound of work that afternoon. If you try, you will probably tire yourself out and be able to do nothing well for the rest of the week. The golden rule is never to increase the time at work more than half an hour a day; do this, and if you're not overtired after a week, try another small increase. Hurrying this up is the recipe for disaster!

Some people find they have reached a plateau and that from month to month their capacity for work doesn't increase. It will be difficult for them to accept that this is permanent, but it's usually wise to do so and to reorganize to meet the challenge. As before, planning the day, delegation, and above all, managing fatigue are the keys to succeeding.

The most important points

People who are recovering from head injury usually have problems with

- Concentration
- Memory
- Organization

- Irritability
- Fatigue
- Emotions

These can occur after mild injuries as well as serious ones. They will need professional help in the early stages and when they are ready to get back to work, from medical people, occupational therapists, and rehabilitation experts.

Don't make an issue of how long it will take to get better. Prophecies are only guesses and if they don't work out you can lose heart.

Fatigue damages all other functions and its management is the most important factor in returning to work.

Families

Never forget that head injury is a family affair. The family has to deal with the shock of the accident, has to take care of their member in the recovery stage, has to understand when there is a change in behaviour, and has to cope with financial problems.

It is essential that everyone concerned realizes this and makes sure that their needs for care and support are met.

Appendix 6
Rivermead symptom checklist

Name: _____

We would like to know whether at the present you suffer from any of the symptoms we list below. Because many of these symptoms occur normally, we would like you to compare yourself as you are now with how you were before the accident.

For each will you please circle the number closest to your answer.

0 = Not experienced at all
1 = Was a problem but no more
2 = A mild problem
3 = A moderate problem
4 = A severe problem

Compared with before the accident, do you now suffer from:

Headaches	0	1	2	3	4
Feelings of dizziness	0	1	2	3	4
Nausea and/or vomiting	0	1	2	3	4
Sensitivity to noise, easily upset by noise	0	1	2	3	4
Poor sleep	0	1	2	3	4
Tiring more easily, fatigue	0	1	2	3	4
Being irritable, easily angered	0	1	2	3	4
Feeling depressed or tearful	0	1	2	3	4
Feeling frustrated or impatient	0	1	2	3	4
Forgetfulness, poor memory	0	1	2	3	4
Poor concentration	0	1	2	3	4
Taking longer to think	0	1	2	3	4
Blurred vision	0	1	2	3	4
Upset by bright light	0	1	2	3	4
Double vision	0	1	2	3	4
Restlessness	0	1	2	3	4

Are you having any other difficulties?

Please describe and rate them as above

1. _____   0   1   2   3   4

2. _____   0   1   2   3   4

Acknowledgements to Rivermead Rehabilitation Centre.

Appendix 7
Glasgow Coma Scale for children

		> 1 year	< 1 year
Eye opening	4	Spontaneous	Spontaneous
	3	To speech	To loud speech
	2	To pain	To pain
	1	None	None
Best motor response	6	Obeys	Normal movement
	5	Localizes pain	Localizes pain
	4	Flexion withdrawal	Flexion withdrawal
	3	Decorticate flexion	Decorticate flexion
	2	Extension	Extension
	1	None	None

		> 5 years	2–5 years	0–23 months
Best 'verbal' response	5	Oriented	Appropriate words, phrases	Smiles, coos, cries appropriately
	4	Confused	Inappropriate words	Cries but consolable
	3	Not appropriate	Cries, screams	Cries, but not consolable
	2	Incomprehensible	Grunts	Grunts, agitated
	1	None	None	None

Index

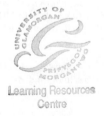